NON-MELANOMA SKIN CANCERS: TARGETED BIOLOGICAL AND SPECIFICALLY DESIGNED THERAPEUTIC AGENTS 2022

Kerry Atkinson MBBS MD DTM&H FRACP FRCP

Consultant Physician

Also by Kerry Atkinson

Medical books

1. Graft-versus-Host Disease. Editors, S Burakoff, H J Deeg, J Ferrara, K Atkinson. Marcel Dekker Inc, New York, 1990.
2. Clinical Bone Marrow Transplantation.First edition. Editor, K Atkinson. Cambridge University Press, Cambridge UK, 1994.
3. The BMT Data Book: A Manual for Bone Marrow and Blood Stem Cell Transplantation. K. Atkinson, Cambridge University Press, Cambridge UK, 1998.
4. Clinical Bone Marrow and Blood Stem Cell Transplantation. Second Edition. Editor, K. Atkinson. Cambridge University Press, Cambridge UK, 2000.
5. Clinical Bone Marrow and Blood Stem Cell Transplantation. Third Edition. Eds, K. Atkinson, R Champlin, J Ritz, M Brenner, P Ljungman and W Fibbe. Cambridge University Press, Cambridge UK, 2004.
6. The BMT Data Book. Second edition. R Munker, HM Lazarus and K. Atkinson, Cambridge University Press, Cambridge UK, 2009.
7. The BMT Data Book: Including Cellular Therapy. Third edition. R Munker, C Hildebrandt, HM Lazarus and K. Atkinson, Cambridge University Press, Cambridge UK. 2013.
8. Hematopoietic Cell Transplants: Concepts, Controversies and Future Directions. Eds HM Lazarus, RP Gale, A Keating, A Bacigalupo, R Munker, K Atkinson, A Syed. Cambridge University Press, Cambridge, UK. 2017.
9. The Biology and Therapeutic Application of Mesenchymal Cells. Ed. K Atkinson. Wiley/Blackwell. 2017
10. Revolutionizing Tropical Medicine. Eds. K Atkinson and D Mabey. Wiley/Blackwell Publishers Inc. 2019.
11. Asthma: Targeted Biological Treatments 2020. Kindle Direct Publishing, 2020. e-book and paperback
12. Atopic Dermatitis: Targeted Biological Treatments 2020. Kindle Direct Publishing, 2020. e-book and paperback
13. Psoriasis: Targeted Biological Treatments 2020. Kindle Direct Publishing, 2020. e-book and paperback
14. Crohn's disease and ulcerative colitis: Targeted Biological Treatments 2020. Kindle Direct Publishing, 2020. e-book and paperback

15. Rheumatoid arthritis, Juvenile Idiopathic Arthritis, Ankylosing spondylitis, Psoriatric Arthritis and Gout: Targeted Biological Treatments 2020. Kindle Direct Publishing, 2020. e-book and paperback
16. Small Cell Lung Cancer: Targeted Biological Treatments 2020. Kindle Direct Publishing, 2020. e-book and paperback
17. Chronic Myeloid Leukemia: Targeted Biological Treatments 2020. Kindle Direct Publishing, 2020. e-book and paperback
18. Melanoma: Targeted Biological Treatments 2020, Kindle Direct Publishing 2020. e-book and paperback
19. Dementia - A Caregiver's Guide. Kindle Direct Publishing 2020. e-book
20. Breast Cancer: Targeted Biological Treatments 2021. Kindle Direct Publishing 2021. e-book and paperback

Natural history/conservation books

21. Bird facts for everyone. K Atkinson. Outskirts Press Inc., Denver, USA. 2014
22. Birds, Birds, Birds. Kindle Direct Publishing 2020. e-book and paperback
23. A Field Guide to the Wild Habitats of Sydney Australia. Kindle Direct Publishing 2021. e-book and paperback
24. Conserving New Zealand's Endangered Species. Kindle Direct Publishing 2021. e-book and paperback
25. Conserving Australia's Endangered Species. Kindle Direct Publishing 2021. e-book and paperback
26. Nature's Wonders: Britain and Ireland. Kindle Direct Publishing 2021. e-book and paperback.

Other

27. Paintings 2019 – 2021. Kindle Direct Publishing 2021. e-book and paperback.

"THE TIMES THEY ARE A-CHANGIN' "

From Bob Dylan's song THE TIMES THEY ARE A-CHANGIN' on his album THE TIMES THEY ARE A-CHANGIN' released by CBS Records in 1964

Nobel Laureate in Literature, 2016

This photograph of Bob Dylan, reproduced here from Wikimedia Commons, is in the public domain. https://commons.wikimedia.org/wiki/File:Bob-Dylan-arrived-at-Arlanda-surrounded-by-twenty-bodyguards-and-assistants-391770740297_(cropped).jpg. This Swedish photograph is in the public domain in Sweden because it is the work is non-artistic (journalistic, etc.) and has been created before 1 January 1970 (SFS 1960:729, § 49a). (1966). (PD 1970)

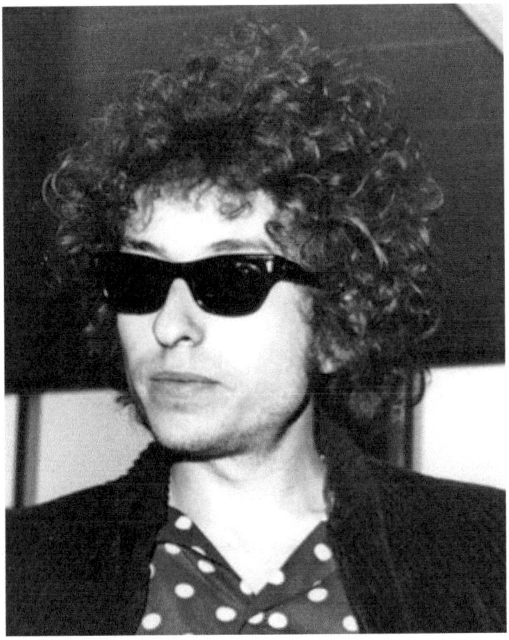

"Old men ought to be explorers
Here and there does not matter
We must be still and still moving
Into another intensity
For a further union, a deeper communion
Through the dark cold and the empty desolation,
The wave cry, the wind cry, the vast waters
Of the petrel and the porpoise. In my end is my beginning."

From Four Quartets. East Coker. By TS Eliot

Nobel Laureate in Literature, 1948.

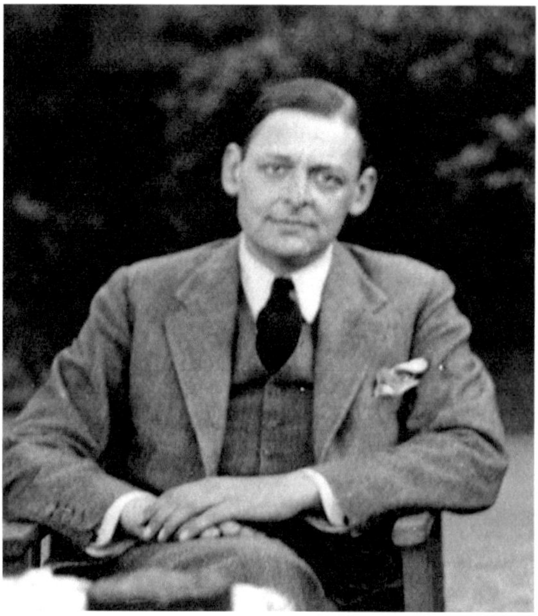

A photograph of TS Eliot taken in 1934. By Thomas Stearns Eliot with his sister and his cousin by Lady Ottoline Morrell.jpg: Lady Ottoline Morrell (1873–1938) derivative work: Octave.H - Thomas Stearns Eliot with his sister and his cousin by Lady Ottoline Morrell.jpg, Public Domain, https://commons.wikimedia.org/w/index.php?curid=7748785. https://en.wikipedia.org/wiki/T._S._Eliot#/media/File:Thomas_Stearns_Eliot_by_Lady_Ottoline_Morrell_(1934).jpg. This work is in the public domain in its country of origin and other countries and areas where the copyright term is the author's life plus 70 years or fewer.

"Ever tried. Ever failed. No matter. Try Again. Fail again. Fail better."
From Worstward Ho by Samuel Beckett. Published by John Calder in 1983

Nobel Laureate in Literature, 1969.

The photograph of Samuel Beckett in 1977, reproduced below from Wikimedia Commons, is in the public domain because its author, Roger Pic has placed it there.

By Roger Pic - Bibliothèque nationale de France, Public Domain, https://commons.wikimedia.org/w/index.php?curid=56362286.

https://en.wikipedia.org/wiki/Samuel_Beckett#/media/File:Samuel_Beckett,_Pic,_1_(cropped).jpg

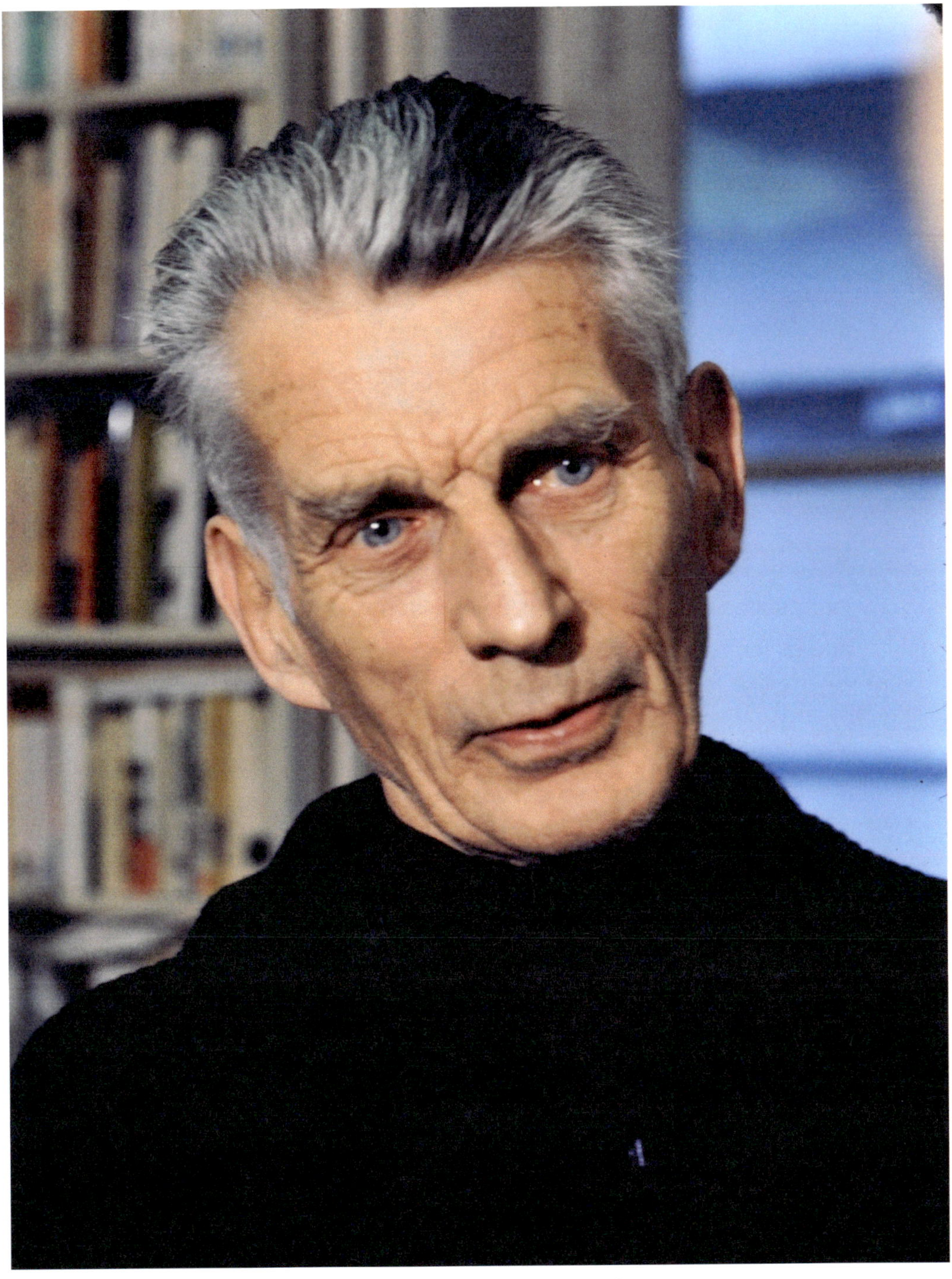

Table of Contents

1. Author's preface

Five major biological revolutions of the second half of the 20th century were

1. The production of monoclonal antibodies
2. The discovery of DNA and how it, RNA and amino acids make proteins
3. Epigenetics and the posttranslational modification of proteins
4. The discovery of cell signalling pathways
5. The cloning of the human genome

Taken together these discoveries in cellular and molecular biology have revealed to scientists appropriate targets for new drugs and the number that have been produced in the last 30 years, and that are still being produced, has hugely enlarged the therapeutic pharmacopeia, producing treatments - even cures - for diseases that were previously untreatable. The majority of these new treatments have been derived because of much more detailed knowledge about how human cells work. They are therefore known as **biological treatments**, often abbreviated to biologics. An example of a biologic is the monoclonal antibody rituximab which reacts specifically with the CD20 antigen present only on B cells, but with no other targets.

In addition, other agents that react specifically with one, or at most, several, targets are **chemically synthesized**: an example is imatinib, which is specific for the tyrosine kinase (TK) domain in abl (the Abelson proto-oncogene), c-kit and PDGF-R (platelet-derived growth factor receptor). Another example is sonedegib, which inhibits activation of the intracellular Hedgehog signalling pathway.

The inclusion of therapeutic agents in this book (and the others in the series) is based on their specificity for a given target. For example, interleukin 2 (IL-2) would not be included since it has a range of biological activities including the proliferation of T cells, the generation of T cell cytotoxic responses and the recall of cytotoxic T cell memory. Likewise interferon-alpha (IFN-α) would not be included since its functions include antiviral activity, antiproliferative activity, NK cell activation, cytokine induction, and interferon-stimulated gene-induction activity. This exclusion applies even though each are made constitutively in the body in response to specific diseases: they are biologic agents, but their targets are broad.

This series of books – one for each disease or disease category - explains what the new treatments are, how they work and how they compare, and interact with, conventional treatment. It is important to state that **no book** in this series makes specific treatment recommendations for any of the diseases covered: such decisions should be initiated and reviewed by an appropriate medical specialist. Much information on each disease is available free of charge from Wikipedia (*wikipedia.org)*, from postgraduate textbooks on each disease and from *UpToDate.com:* the latter website gives information for patients and caregivers free of charge but a subscription is required for more detailed information (uptodate.com). **Rather**, the purpose of this series of books is to give information on newly developed biological and specifically designed treatments and their mechanism of action, enabling hopefully the reader to get a handle on these extensive additions to the medical pharmacopeia.

This book includes biological targeted treatments for non-melanoma skin cancers approved for therapeutic use in the United States of America (USA) by the USA Food and Drug Administration (FDA). A distinction is sometimes made between monoclonal antibodies (the mabs) as "immunotherapy", the small specifically designed inhibitory molecules (the nibs) and the receptor blocking agents (the cepts) – the latter sometimes known as decoy receptors. However, since each category of drug has been developed from the comprehensive knowledge of human cell biology discovered over the past seven decades, and as each drug in each category is exquisitely targeted to a specific epitope on a cell surface protein (the mabs), the inhibition of a specific intracellular enzyme process (the nibs), or the blocking of a specific cell surface receptor (the cepts) I prefer to combine the mabs, the nibs and the cepts in the single category of targeted biological treatments. An example from each category are rituximab, imatinib and etanercept.

There is now a fourth type of biological targeted therapeutic agents – chimeric antigen receptor (CAR) T cells. The first such agent – tisagenlecleucel – was approved by the USA FDA in 2018 for use in people with acute lymphoblastic leukemia. CAR T cells are an innovative cellular immunotherapeutic approach that involves genetic modification of autologous T cells to express CAR targeting tumor antigen/s as well as a component of the T cell activation pathway – the CD3 zeta chain. T-cell surface glycoprotein CD3 zeta chain, also known as T-cell receptor T3 zeta chain or CD247, together with T-cell receptor alpha/beta and gamma/delta heterodimers and CD3-gamma, -delta, and -epsilon, forms the T-cell receptor-CD3 complex. The zeta chain plays an important role in coupling antigen recognition to several intracellular signal-transduction pathways. There are now three CAR T cell therapeutics that are FDA-approved for people with aggressive lymphomas.

I have included in this book a fifth type of biological targeted agents – sonidegib and vismodegib – both of which specifically target the intracellular Hedgehog pathway and are now both FDA-approved for treatment of basal cell carcinoma of the skin

These new drug discovery phenomenon is a therapeutic tsunami which shows no sign of slowing. The pharmcopiea has increased enormously and all medical students should consider doing a Master's degree or a PhD in molecular biology. It is only by working in a cellular or molecular biology laboratory (usually combined) that one can really understand how each of these new medications work.

It should be noted that all text on each individual drug is taken directly from the USA FDA's product approval label for that drug, including the drug's generic name, its brand name, the indications for which it is approved, its mechanism of action, boxed warnings and other details on warnings, precautions, adverse events and specific patient populations. These are all in the public domain and can be accessed at https://www.accessdata.fda.gov/scripts/cder/daf/.

Only the prodct label information was take from the FDA. All images and illustrations were taken from a variety of sources. Most of these are in the public domain, but some are licensed by a Creative Commons license. Each image carries the legend written by the creator of the image as well as full attribution details required by the creator. No images were used from the FDA's product approval label for each drug.

A side-effect seen with a number of biologic agents are immune-mediated syndromes. To distinguish them from each other, a brief summary of each is given in Appendices C to F. Additionally, Appendix A lists the Child-Pugh grading system for hepatic impairment and Appendix B lists the internationally accepted classification of both clinical and laboratory adverse events published by the USA Department of Health and Human Services

I would like to acknowledge the help that I received from Jim Severino in designing the cover for this book and for uploading it for me to Kindle Direct Publishing.

2. Introduction to the new targeted biologic and specifically designed therapeutic agents

Biologic sand biosimilars

A **biosimilar** is a biologic medical product highly similar to another already approved biological medicine. Biosimilars are approved according to the same standards of pharmaceutical quality, safety and efficacy that apply to all biological medicines. Biosimilars are officially approved versions of original "innovator" products and can be manufactured when the original product's patent expires. Reference to the innovator product is an integral component of the approval.

It should be noted (as in the text below) that many, if not all, of these new treatments have many, and often serious side-effects, including adverse interactions when combined with other drugs.

Finally, most of these new treatments are extremely expensive ("financial toxicity"), which renders both access to them, and sometimes compliance with them, impossible or suboptimal.

Monoclonal antibodies (mabs)

Background

In 1975, Georges Köhler and César Milstein in the UK succeeded in producing a hybridoma by making fusions of murine myeloma cell lines with murine B cells. This immortalized hybridoma could produce antibodies specific for known antigens. In 1985 the FDA approved the first fully licensed Mab (Muromonab, anti-CD3 for use in preventing kidney transplant rejection. Muromonab was produced using only murine cells and thus the antibodies produced were wholly murine. Subsequently, to decrease immunogenicity of murine antibodies, chimeric antibodies were created in which the constant (Fc) portion of the antibody was human, while the variable (Fab-binding) regions remained of murine origin. After this, humanized mabs were produced in which the framework and constant regions were human, while the hypervariable region remained of murine origin. After this, fully human mabs were produced, lacking any murine component. Finally, it is now possible to produce mabs solely using recombinant DNA technology.

Mabs may be used in many different ways. This is illustrated in Figure 1 for mabs that are developed for the treatment of disease.

Figure 1

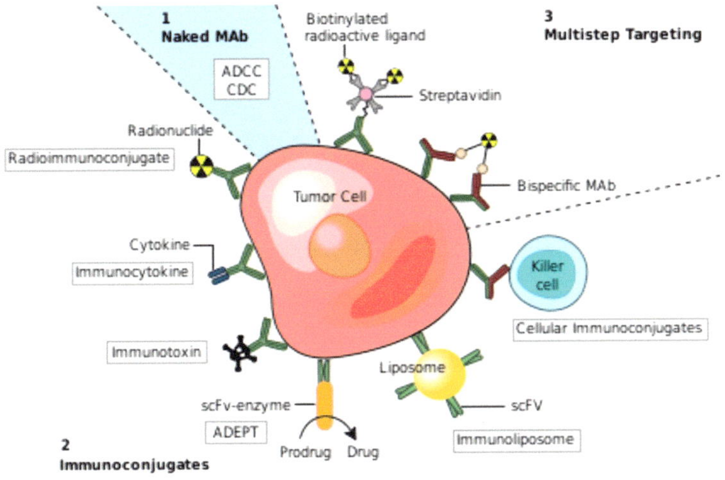

Abbreviations used in Figure 1: antibody directed enzyme prodrug therapy; ADCC: antibody-dependent cell-mediated cytotoxicity; CDC: complement-dependent cytotoxicity; MAb, monoclonal antibody; scFv, single-chain Fv fragment

Nomenclature convention for monoclonal antibodies

Murine mabs have the prefix –o- before mab; eg, abagovomab. (Note: the first murine mab approved by the FDA (Muromonab, anti-CD3) deviated from this nomenclature which was not in place at the time of its approval).

Chimeric mabs have the prefix –xi- before mab; eg, basilixumab

Humanized mabs have the prefix –zu- before mab; eg, trastuzumab

Human mabs have the prefix –u- before mab; eg, atinumab

Examples of these new agents and their mechanism of action in the treatment of non-malignant diseases

Monoclonal antibodies

- Receptor antagonists – eg, dapulimab (anti IL-4 and anti-IL13 signalling) in atopic dermatitis
- Apoptosis (programmed cell death) inducers – eg, rituximab in B cell-mediated autoimmune diseases
- Immune pathway inhibitors – eg, dipilumab for IL-4 and IL-13 signalling in atopic dermatitis, infliximab and adalimumab for TNF inhibition in psoriasis; secukinumab for IL-17 inhibition in psoriasis; ustekinumab for IL-12/Th1 inhibition and IL-23/ILTh17 inhibition in psoriasis; ixekizumab as an anti-IL17A agent in psoriasis; brodalumab as an anti-IL-7 receptor antagonist in psoriasis
- TNF pathway antagonists – eg, adalimumab for psoriasis
- Integrin pathway blockers – eg, natalizumab for Crohn's disease
- Rank ligand inhibitor – eg, denosumab for targeted treatment of postmenopausal women with osteoporosis at high risk for fracture
- Angiogenesis inhibitors – eg, ranibizumab for macular degeneration

- Dabigatran binder – eg, idarucizumab for bleeding due to dabigatran administration
- Proprotein convertase subtilisin kexin type 9 (PCSK9) inhibitor – eg, alirocumab and evolocumab for dyslipidemias
- Bi-specific antibodies – eg, emicizumab-kxwh for hemophilia A
- Monoclonal antibody-delivered toxins or drugs

A list of all monoclonal antibodies and receptor blocking agents that are USA FDA-approved for therapeutic use for either non-malignant disease, malignant disease or both malignant and and non-malignant disease is shown in Table 1 (as of December 2020).

Table1

Generic name/brand name/type of mab	**Target**	**FDA-approved indication/s**
Abciximab/ ReoPro/ chimeric fab fragment	GPIIb/IIIa	Percutaneous coronary intervention for the prevention of cardiac ischemic complications in patients undergoing percutaneous coronary intervention or in patients with unstable angina not responding to conventional medical therapy when percutaneous coronary intervention is planned within 24 hours
Adalimumab/ Humira/ fully human	TNF	Rheumatoid arthritis (RA), juvenile idiopathic arthritis (JIA), ankylosing spondylitis (AS), psoriatric arthrtitis, Crohn's disease[1], ulcerative colitis, plaque psoriasis, hidradenitis suppura[a], non-infectious uveitis
Adalimumab-abdm/Cyltezo/ fully human, biosimilar	TNF	RA, JIA, AS, psoriatric arthritis, Crohn's disease[1], ulcerative colitis, plaque psoriasis,
Adalimumab-atto/Amjevita/ fully human, biosimilar	TNF	RA, JIA, AS, psoriatric arthritis, Crohn's disease[1], ulcerative colitis, plaque psoriasis
Ado-trastuzumab Emtasine/ Kadcyla/	HER2	HER2-positive, metastatic breast cancer who previously received trastuzumab and a taxane, separately or in combination. Patients should have either:

humanized antibody-microtubule inhibitor conjugate		• received prior therapy for metastatic disease, or • developed disease recurrence during or within six months of completing adjuvant therapy. • the adjuvant treatment of patients with HER2-positive early breast cancer who have residual invasive disease after neoadjuvant taxane and trastuzumab-based treatment.
Alemtuzumab/ Campath, Lemtrada/ humanized	CD52	Relapsing forms of multiple sclerosis (MS) (previously approved for chronic lymphocytic leukemia but now withdrawn by its manufacturer for this indication in order to optimize its launch for treatment of MS)
Alirocumab/ Praluent/fully human	PCSK9 (proprotein convertase subtilisin kexin type 9) inhibitor	Adjunct to diet and maximally tolerated statin therapy for the treatment of adults with heterozygous familial hypercholesterolemia or clinical atherosclerotic cardiovascular disease, who require additional lowering of LDL-cholesterol (LDL-C).
Ansuvimab-zykl / EBANGA™		Treatment of infection caused by Zaire ebolavirus in adult and pediatric patients, including neonates born to a mother who is RT-PCR positive for Zaire ebolavirus infection.
Atezolizumab/ Tecentriq/ humanized	Programmed death ligand 1 (PD-L1)	1. Urothelial carcinoma for the treatment of adult patients with locally advanced or metastatic urothelial carcinoma who are not eligible for cisplatin-containing chemotherapy and whose tumors express PD-L1 or who are not eligible for any platinum-containing chemotherapy regardless of PD-L1 status, or who have disease progression during or following any platinum-containing chemotherapy, or within 12 months of neoadjuvant or adjuvant chemotherapy. This indication is approved under accelerated approval based on tumor response rate and duration of response. Continued approval for this indication may be contingent upon verification and description of clinical benefit in a confirmatory trial(s). 2. Non-small cell lung ancer (NSCLC) in combination with bevacizumab, paclitaxel, and carboplatin for the firstline treatment, of adult patients with metastatic non-squamous NSCLC with no EGFR or ALK genomic tumor aberrations or for the treatment of adult patients with metastatic NSCLC who have disease progression during or following platinum-containing chemotherapy. Patients with EGFR or ALK genomic tumor aberrations should have disease progression on FDA-approved therapy for NSCLC harboring these aberrations prior to receiving TECENTRIQ. 2. Triple-negative breast cancer (TNBC) in combination with paclitaxel for the treatment of adult patients with unresectable locally advanced or metastatic TNBC whose tumors express PD-L1. This indication is approved under accelerated approval based on progression-free survival. Continued approval for this indication may be contingent upon verification and description of clinical benefit in a confirmatory trial(s).
Atoltivimab,	INMAZEB is a	Zaire ebolavirus in adult and pediatric patients, including

maftivimab, and odesivimab-ebgn) injection/ INMAZEB™	combination of three recombinant human IgG1κ monoclonal antibodies each targeting the Zaire ebolavirus glycoprotein (GP). Zaire ebolavirus encodes a sole envelope protein, the glycoprotein, which mediates virus attachment and membrane fusion with the host cell membranes. In addition, GP is expressed on the surface of Zaire ebolavirus infected host cells making it a target for antibodies that can mediate killing of these cells by antibody-dependent cellular cytotoxicity and/or other effector functions. The 3 antibodies that make up the combination can bind the GP simultaneously	neonates born to a mother who is RT-PCR positive for Zaire ebolavirus infection.
Avelumab/ Bavencio/ fully human	PD-L1	1. Adult and pediatric patients 12 years and older with metastatic Merkel cell carcinoma[2a] 2. Patients with locally advanced or metastatic urothelial carcinoma who have disease progression during or following platinum-containing chemotherapy or who have disease progression within 12 months of neoadjuvant or adjuvant treatment with platinum-containing chemotherapy[a]. 3. First-line treatment, in combination with axitinib, of patients with advanced renal cell carcinoma [a]Continued approval for this indication may be contingent upon verification and description of clinical benefit in confirmatory trials
Basiliximab/ Simulect/ chimeric	IL-2 receptor alpha chain (IL-2Rα) blocker	Prophylaxis of acute organ rejection in patients receiving renal transplantation when used as part of an immunosuppressive regimen that includes cyclosporine and corticosteroids
Belimumab/	B lymphocyte	Active, autoantibody-positive, systemic lupus

Benlysta/fully human	stimulator (BLyS) -specific inhibitor	erythematosus (SLE) in adults who are receiving standard therapy
Benralizumab/ Fasenra/ humanized	Interleukin-5 receptor-α	For the add-on maintenance treatment of patients with severe asthma aged 12 years and older, and with an eosinophilic phenotype
Bevacizumab/ Avastin/ humanized	Vascular endothelial growth factor (VEGF)-specific angiogenesis	1. Metastatic colorectal cancer, with intravenous 5-fluorouracil–based chemotherapy for first- or second-line treatment. 2. Non-squamous non-small cell lung cancer, with carboplatin and paclitaxel for first line treatment of unresectable, locally advanced, recurrent or metastatic disease. 3. Metastatic breast cancer, with paclitaxel for treatment of patients who have not received chemotherapy for metastatic HER2-negative breast cancer. 4.Glioblastoma, as a single agent for adult patients with progressive disease following prior therapy 5. Metastatic renal cell carcinoma with interferon-α
Bevacizumab-awwb/Mvasi/ humanized biosimilar	VEGF	1. Metastatic colorectal cancer, in combination with intravenous fluorouracil-based chemotherapy for first- or second-line treatment. 2. Metastatic colorectal cancer, in combination with fluoropyrimidine-irinotecan- or fluoropyrimidine-oxaliplatin-based chemotherapy for second-line treatment in patients who have progressed on a first-line bevacizumab product-containing regimen. 3. Unresectable, locally advanced, recurrent or metastatic non-squamous non-small cell lung cancer, in combination with carboplatin and paclitaxel for first-line treatment. 4. Recurrent glioblastoma in adults. 5. Metastatic renal cell carcinoma in combination with interferon-α. 6. Persistent, recurrent, or metastatic cervical cancer, in combination with paclitaxel and cisplatin, or paclitaxel and topotecan.
Bevlotuxumab/ Zinplava/fully human	Clostridium difficile toxin	Reduction of recurrence of Clostridium difficile infection (CDI) in patients 18 years of age or older who are receiving antibacterial drug treatment of CDI and are at a high risk for CDI recurrence.
Belantamab mafodotin-blmf/ BLENREP Antibody-drug conjugate	Myeloma	Belantamab mafodotin-blmf is an antibody-drug conjugate (ADC). The antibody component is an afucosylated IgG1 directed against BCMA, a protein expressed on normal B lymphocytes and multiple myeloma cells. The small molecule component is MMAF, a microtubule inhibitor. Upon binding to BCMA, belantamab mafodotin-blmf is internalized followed by release of MMAF via proteolytic cleavage. The released MMAF intracellularly disrupts the microtubule network, leading to cell cycle arrest and apoptosis. Belantamab mafodotin-blmf had antitumor activity in multiple myeloma cells and mediated killing of

		tumor cells through MMAF-induced apoptosis, as well as by tumor cell lysis through antibody-dependent cellular cytotoxicity (ADCC) and antibody-dependent cellular phagocytosis (ADCP).
Blinatumomab/ Blincyto/ murine bispecific CD19-directed CD3 T cell engager	CD19	1. B cell precursor acute lymphoblastic leukemia (ALL) in first or second complete remission with minimal residual disease (MRD) greater than or equal to 0.1%. This indication is approved under accelerated approval based on MRD response rate and hematological relapse-free survival. Continued approval for this indication may be contingent upon verification and description of clinical benefit in the confirmatory trials. 2. Relapsed or refractory B cell precursor acute lymphoblastic leukemia
Brentuximab vedotin/ Adcetris/ chimeric, antibody-drug conjugate	CD30	1.Classical Hodgkin lymphoma[3] (cHL) at high risk of relapse or progression as post autologous hematopoietic stem cell transplantation (auto-HSCT) consolidation 2.Classical Hodgkin lymphoma after failure of auto-HSCT or after failure of at least two prior multi-agent chemotherapy regimens in patients who are not auto-HSCT candidates 3. Systemic anaplastic large cell lymphoma (sALCL) after failure of at least one prior multi-agent chemotherapy regimen. Accelerated approval was granted for the sALCL indication based on overall response rate. Continued approval for this indication may be contingent upon verification and description of clinical benefit in confirmatory trials. 4. Primary cutaneous anaplastic large cell lymphoma (pcALCL) or CD30 expressing mycosis fungoides who have received prior systemic therapy
Brodalumab/ Siliq/chimeric	!L-17 receptor	Moderate to severe plaque psoriasis in adult patients who are candidates for systemic therapy or phototherapy and have failed to respond or have lost response to other systemic therapies.
Burosumab-twza/Crysvita/ fully human	Fibroblast growth factor (FGF)23	X-linked hypophosphatemia (XLH) in adult and pediatric patients 6 months of age and older
Canakinuab/ Ilaris/fully human	IL-1β	Cryopyrin-associated periodic syndromes (CAPS), in adults and children 4 years of age and older including familial cold autoinflammatory syndrome (FCAS) and Muckle-Wells Syndrome (MWS)
Capromab pendetide/ Prosta-Scint/ murine radio-labelled (Indium [111])	Prostate-specific membrane antigen (PSMA)	1. A diagnostic imaging agent in newly-diagnosed patients with biopsy-proven prostate cancer, thought to be clinically-localized after standard diagnostic evaluation (e.g. chest x-ray, bone scan, CT scan, or MRI), who are at high-risk for pelvic lymph node metastases 2. A diagnostic imaging agent in post-prostatectomy patients with a rising PSA leveland a negative or equivocal standard metastatic evaluation in whom there is

		a high clinical suspicion of occult metastatic disease.
Certolizumab Pegol/Cimzia/ humanized (pegylated for longer duration of action)	TNF	1.Crohn's disease 2.Rheumatoid arthritis 3.Psoriatic arthritis 4.Ankylosing spondylitis
Cetuximab/ Erbitux/ chimeric	Epidermal growth factor (EGF) receptor	1.Head and neck cancer Locally or regionally advanced squamous cell carcinoma of the head and neck in combination with radiation therapy. Recurrent loco-regional disease or metastatic squamous cell carcinoma of the head and neck in combination with platinum-based therapy with 5-FU. Recurrent or metastatic squamous cell carcinoma of the head and neck progressing after platinum-based therapy. 2.Colorectal cancer As a single agent, EGFR-expressing metastatic colorectal cancer after failure of both irinotecan- and oxaliplatin-based regimens or in patients who are intolerant to irinotecan-based regimens. In combination with irinotecan, EGFR-expressing metastatic colorectal carcinoma in patients who are refractory to irinotecan-based chemotherapy.
Cemiplimab/ Libtayo/ humanized	PD-1	Metastatic cutaneous squamous cell carcinoma (CSCC) or locally advanced CSCC who are not candidates for curative surgery or curative radiation.
Daclizumab/ Zenapax/ humanized	IL-2 receptor-α	Prophylaxis of acute organ rejection in patients receiving renal transplants. It is used as part of an immunosuppressive regimen that includes cyclosporine and corticosteroids.
Naxitamab-gqgk/ Danyelza	Naxitamab-gqgk binds to the glycolipid GD2. GD2 is a disialoganglioside that is overexpress-ed on neuroblasto-ma cells and other cells of neuroectod-ermal origin, including the central nervous system and peripheral nerves. In vitro, naxitamab-gqgk was able to bind to cell surface GD2 and induce	DANYELZA is a GD2-binding monoclonal antibody indicated, in combination with granulocyte-macrophage colony-stimulating factor (GMCSF), for the treatment of pediatric patients 1 year of age and older and adult patients with relapsed or refractory high-risk neuroblastoma in the bone or bone marrow who have demonstrated a partial response, minor response, or stable disease to prior therapy

	complement-dependent cytotoxicity (CDC) and antibody dependent- cell-mediated cytotoxicity (ADCC).	
Darzalex/ Zinbryta/ humanized	IL-2 receptor	Relapsing forms of multiple sclerosis (MS). Because of its safety profile, the use of ZINBRYTA should generally be reserved for patients who have had an inadequate response to two or more drugs indicated for the treatment of MS.
Daratumumab/ Darzalex/fully human	CD38	Multiple myeloma 1.In combination with lenalidomide and dexamethasone in newly diagnosed patients who are ineligible for autologous stem cell transplant and in patients with relapsed or refractory multiple myeloma who have received at least one prior therapy 2.In combination with bortezomib, melphalan and prednisone in newly diagnosed patients who are ineligible for autologous stem cell transplant 3.In combination with bortezomib and dexamethasone in patients who have received at least one prior therapy 4.In combination with pomalidomide and dexamethasone in patients who have received at least two prior therapies including lenalidomide and a proteasome inhibitor 5. As monotherapy, in patients who have received at least three prior lines of therapy including a proteasome inhibitor (PI) and an immunomodulatory agent or who are double-refractory to a PI and an immunomodulatory agent.
Denosumab/ Prolia/fully human	Receptor activator of nuclear factor kappa-B ligand (RANKL)	1.Postmenopausal women with osteoporosis at high risk for fracture 2.Treatment to increase bone mass in men at high risk for fracture receiving androgen deprivation therapy for non-metastatic prostate cancer 3.Treatment to increase bone mass in women at high risk for fracture receiving adjuvant aromatase inhibitor therapy for breast cancer
Denosumab/ Xgeva/fully human	RANKL	1.Prevention of skeletal-related events in patients with multiple myeloma and in patients with bone metastases from solid tumors 2.Treatment of adults and skeletally mature adolescents with giant cell tumor of bone that is unresectable or where surgical resection is likely to result in severe morbidity 3.Treatment of hypercalcemia of malignancy refractory to bisphosphonate therapy
Dinutuximab/ Unituxin/	GD2 (a disialo-	In combination with granulocyte-macrophage colony-stimulating factor (GM-CSF), interleukin-2 (IL-2), and 13-

chimeric	ganglioside)	cis-retinoic acid (RA), for the treatment of pediatric patients with high-risk neuroblastoma who achieve at least a partial response to prior first-line multiagent, multimodality therapy
Dupilumab/ Dupixent/fully human	IL-4 receptor-α (IL 4RA)	1. For patients aged 12 years and older with moderate-to-severe atopic dermatitis whose disease is not adequately controlled with topical prescription therapies or when those therapies are not advisable. 2. As an add-on maintenance treatment in patients with moderate-to-severe asthma aged 12 years and older with an eosinophilic phenotype or with oral corticosteroid-dependent asthma. 3. As an add-on maintenance treatment in adult patients with inadequately controlled chronic rhinosinusitis with nasal polyposis (CRSwNP).
Durvalumab/ Imfinzi/fully human	PD-L1	1.Locally advanced or metastatic urothelial carcinoma who have disease progression during or following platinum-containing chemotherapy or who have disease or progression within 12 months of neoadjuvant or adjuvant treatment with platinum-containing chemotherapy 2. Unresectable, stage III non-small cell lung cancer (NSCLC) whose disease has not progressed following concurrent platinum-based chemotherapy and radiation therapy.
Eculizumab/ Solaris/ humanized	Complement component 5	1.Paroxysmal nocturnal hemoglobinuria (PNH) to reduce hemolysis 2.Atypical hemolytic uremic syndrome (aHUS) to inhibit complement-mediated thrombotic microangiopathy
Elotuzumab/ Empliciti/ humanized	Signalling lymphocytic activation molecule family (SLAMF7, CD319)	In combination with lenalidomide and dexamethasone for the treatment of multiple myeloma who have received one to three prior therapies.
Emicizumab-kxwh/ Hemlibra/ humanized bispecific	Factor IXa, Factor X (bridges activated factor IX and factor X to restore the function of missing activated factor VIII that is needed for effective hemostasis)	Routine prophylaxis to prevent or reduce the frequency of bleeding episodes in adult and pediatric patients ages newborn and older with hemophilia A (congenital factor VIII deficiency) with or without factor VIII inhibitors.
Eptinezumab-jjmr/VYEPTI/ humanized	CGRP	VYEPTI is a calcitonin gene-related peptide antagonist indicated for the preventive treatment of migraine in adults. Eptinezumab-jjmr is a humanized monoclonal antibody that binds to calcitonin gene-related peptide (CGRP) ligand and blocks its binding to the receptor

Erenumab-aooe/Aimovig/ fully human	Calcitonin gene-related peptide receptor (CGRP receptor)	Antagonist indicated for the preventive treatment of migraine in adults
Evolocumab/ Repatha/fully human	Proprotein convertase subtilisin kexin type 9 (PCSK9)	1. To reduce the risk of myocardial infarction, stroke, and coronary revascularization in adults with established cardiovascular disease. 2. As an adjunct to diet, alone or in combination with other lipid-lowering therapies (e.g., statins, ezetimibe), for treatment of adults with primary hyperlipidemia (including heterozygous familial hypercholesterolemia) to reduce low-density lipoprotein cholesterol (LDL-C). 3. As an adjunct to diet and other LDL-lowering therapies (e.g., statins, ezetimibe, LDL apheresis) in patients with homozygous familial hypercholesterolemia (HoFH) who require additional lowering of LDL-C.
Gemtuzumab ozogamicin/ Mylotarg/ humanized antibody-drug conjugate (N-acetyl gamma calichea-micin)	CD33	1.Newly-diagnosed CD33-positive acute myeloid leukemia (AML) in adults 2.Relapsed or refractory CD33-positive AML in adults and in pediatric patients 2 years and older
Golimumab/ Simponi/fully human	TNF	1.Moderately to severely active RA in adults, in combination with methotrexate 2.Active psoriatic arthritis in adults, alone or in combination with methotrexate 3.Active AS in adults
Golimumab/ Simponi Aria/ fully human	TNF	1.Moderately to severely RA in combination with methotrexate 2.Active psoriatic arthritis 3.Active AS
Guselkumab/ Tremfya/fully human	IL-23	Adult patients with moderate-to-severe plaque psoriasis who are candidates for systemic therapy or phototherapy
Ibalizumab-uiyk/Trogarzo/ humanized	CD4	In combination with other antiretroviral(s), for the treatment of human immunodeficiency virus type 1 (HIV-1) infection in heavily treatment-experienced adults with multidrug resistant HIV-1 infection failing their current antiretroviral regimen
Ibritumomab tiuxetan/ Zevalin/ murine radio-	CD20	1.Relapsed or refractory, low-grade or follicular B cell non-Hodgkin's lymphoma 2. Previously untreated follicular B cell non-Hodgkin lymphoma who achieve a partial or complete response to

immunoconjug-ate (the chelate tiuxetan, which tightly binds to Indium^{111} or Ytrium^{90}, is covalently linked to ibritumomab. The beta emission from Y^{90} induces cellular damage by the formation of free radicals in the target and neighboring cells)		first-line chemotherapy
Idarucizumab/ Praxbind/ humanized fab fragment	Dabigatran (Pradaxa)	Patients treated with Pradaxa® when reversal of the anticoagulant effects of dabigatran is needed: 1. For emergency surgery/urgent procedures 2. In life-threatening or uncontrolled bleeding. This indication is approved under accelerated approval based on a reduction in unbound dabigatran and normalization of coagulation parameters in healthy volunteers. Continued approval for this indication may be contingent upon the results of an ongoing cohort case series study.
Inebilizumab-cdon/ UPLIZNATM	CD19	UPLIZNA is a CD19-directed cytolytic antibody indicated for the treatment of neuromyelitis optica spectrum disorder (NMOSD) in adult patients who are anti-aquaporin-4 (AQP4) antibody positive.
Infliximab/ Remicade/ chimeric	TNF-α	1. Crohn's disease for reducing signs and symptoms and inducing and maintaining clinical remission in adult patients with moderately to severely active disease who have had an inadequate response to conventional therapy. For reducing the number of draining enterocutaneous and rectovaginal fistulas and maintaining fistula closure in adult patients with fistulizing disease. 2. Pediatric Crohn's disease for reducing signs and symptoms and inducing and maintaining clinical remission in pediatric patients with moderately to severely active disease who have had an inadequate response to conventional therapy. 3.Ulcerative colitis for reducing signs and symptoms, inducing and maintaining clinical remission and mucosal healing, and eliminating corticosteroid use in adult patients with moderately to severely active disease who have had an inadequate response to conventional

		therapy. 4. Pediatric ulcerative colitis for reducing signs and symptoms and inducing and maintaining clinical remission in pediatric patients with moderately to severely active disease who have had an inadequate response to conventional therapy. 5. Rheumatoid arthritis in combination with methotrexate for reducing signs and symptoms, inhibiting the progression of structural damage, and improving physical function in patients with moderately to severely active disease. 6. Ankylosing spondylitis for reducing signs and symptoms in patients with active disease. 7. Psoriatic arthritis for reducing signs and symptoms of active arthritis, inhibiting the progression of structural damage, and improving physical function. 8. Plaque psoriasis for treatment of adult patients with chronic severe (i.e., extensive and /or disabling) plaque psoriasis who are candidates for systemic therapy and when other systemic therapies are medically less appropriate.
Infliximab-abda/Renflexis /chimeric biosimilar	TNF-α	Similar to Remicade: see https://www.accessdata.fda.gov/drugsatfda_docs/label/2017/761054orig1s000lbl.pdf
Infliximab-dyyb/Inflectra/ chimeric biosimilar	TNF-α	Similar to Remicade. See https://www.accessdata.fda.gov/drugsatfda_docs/label/2016/125544s000lbl.pdf
Infliximab-qbtx/Ixifi chimeric biosimilar	TNF-α	Similar to Remicade. See https://www.accessdata.fda.gov/drugsatfda_docs/label/2017/761072s000lbl.pdf
Inotuzumab ozogamicin/ Besponsa/ humanized; antibody-drug conjugate (N-acetyl gamma calicheamicin)	CD22	Adults with relapsed or refractory B cell precursor acute lymphoblastic leukemia (ALL)
Ipilimomab/ Yervoy/fully human	CTLA-4	Melanoma • Treatment of unresectable or metastatic melanoma in adults and pediatric patients (12 years and older). • Adjuvant treatment of patients with cutaneous melanoma with pathologic involvement of regional lymph nodes of more than 1 mm who have undergone complete resection, including total

		lymphadenectomy. Renal Cell Carcinoma (RCC) • Treatment of patients with intermediate or poor-risk, previously untreated advanced renal cell carcinoma, in combination with nivolumab. Colorectal Cancer • Treatment of adult and pediatric patients 12 years of age and older with microsatellite instability-high (MSI-H) or mismatch repair deficient (dMMR) metastatic colorectal cancer that has progressed following treatment with a fluoropyrimidine, oxaliplatin, and irinotecan, in combination with nivolumab. • This indication is approved under accelerated approval based on overall response rate and duration of response. Continued approval for this indication may be contingent upon verification and description of clinical benefit in confirmatory trials. Hepatocellular Carcinoma • Treatment of patients with hepatocellular carcinoma who have been previously treated with sorafenib, in combination with nivolumab. This indication is approved under accelerated approval based on overall response rate and duration of response. Continued approval for this indication may be contingent upon verification and description of clinical benefit in confirmatory trials. Non-Small Cell Lung Cancer (NSCLC) • Treatment of adult patients with metastatic non-small cell lung cancer expressing PD-L1 (≥1%) as determined by an FDA-approved test, with no EGFR or ALK genomic tumor aberrations, as first-line treatment in combination with nivolumab. • Treatment of adult patients with metastatic or recurrent non-small cell lung cancer with no EGFR or ALK genomic tumor aberrations as first-line treatment, in combination with ipilimumab and 2 cycles of platinum-doublet chemotherapy
Ixekizumab/ Taltz/ humanized	IL-17A antagonist (often referred to as IL-17)	Adults with 1. Moderate-to-severe plaque psoriasis who are candidates for systemic therapy or phototherapy. 2. Active psoriatic arthritis. 3. Active ankylosing spondylitis
Margetuximab-cmkb/ Margenza	Her2/neu	Margenza is a HER2/neu receptor antagonist indicated, in combination with chemotherapy, for the treatment of adult patients with metastatic HER2 positive breast cancer who have received two or more prior anti-HER2 regimens, at

		least one of which was for metastatic disease
Mepolizumab/ Nucala/ humanized	IL-5	Add-on maintenance treatment of patients with severe asthma aged 12 years and older, and with an eosinophilic phenotype
Mogamuliz-umab/ Poteligeo/ humanized	CCR4 (CC chemo-kines have 2 adjacent cysteine near their amino terminus)	Adult patients with relapsed or refractory mycosis fungoides or Sézary syndrome after at least one prior systemic therapy
Moxetumomab pasudotox Lumoxiti/ murine antibody-drug conjugate. (the toxin called PE38, is a 38kDa fragment of Pseudomonas exotoxin A.	CD22	Adult patients with relapsed or refractory hairy cell leukemia (HCL) who received at least two prior systemic therapies, including treatment with a purine nucleoside analog (PNA)
Natalizumab/ Tysabri/ humanized	α4 integrin	1. Multiple sclerosis (MS): as monotherapy for the treatment of patients with relapsing forms of multiple sclerosis to delay the accumulation of physical disability and reduce the frequency of clinical exacerbations. TYSABRI is generally recommended for patients who have had an inadequate response to, or are unable to tolerate, an alternate MS therapy. 2.Crohn's disease: inducing and maintaining clinical response and remission in adult patients with moderately to severely active Crohn's disease with evidence of inflammation who have had an inadequate response to, or are unable to tolerate, conventional Crohn's disease therapies and inhibitors of TNF-α.
Necitumumab/ Portrazza/ fully human	EGFR	In combination with gemcitabine and cisplatin, for first-line treatment of patients with metastatic squamous non-small cell lung cancer
Nivolumab/ Opdivo/ fully human	PD-1	Melanoma • patients with unresectable or metastatic melanoma, as a single agent or in combination with ipilimumab • patients with melanoma with lymph node involvement or metastatic disease who have undergone complete resection, in the adjuvant setting. Non-Small Cell Lung Cancer (NSCLC) • adult patients with metastatic non-small cell lung cancer expressing PD-L1 (≥1%) as determined by an FDA-approved test, with no EGFR or ALK genomic tumor aberrations, as first-line treatment in combination with ipilimumab.

		• adult patients with metastatic or recurrent non-small cell lung cancer with no EGFR or ALK genomic tumor aberrations as first-line treatment, in combination with ipilimumab and 2 cycles of platinum-doublet chemotherapy. • patients with metastatic non-small cell lung cancer and progression on or after platinum-based chemotherapy. Patients with EGFR or ALK genomic tumor aberrations should have disease progression on FDA-approved therapy for these aberrations prior to receiving OPDIVO . Malignant Pleural Mesothelioma • adult patients with unresectable malignant pleural mesothelioma, as first-line treatment in combination with ipilimumab. Renal Cell Carcinoma (RCC) • patients with intermediate or poor risk advanced renal cell carcinoma, as a first-line treatment in combination with ipilimumab. • patients with advanced renal cell carcinoma, as a first-line treatment in combination with cabozantinib. • patients with advanced renal cell carcinoma who have received prior antiangiogenic therapy. Classical Hodgkin Lymphoma (cHL) • adult patients with classical Hodgkin lymphoma that has relapsed or progressed after • autologous hematopoietic stem cell transplantation (HSCT) and brentuximab vedotin, or • 3 or more lines of systemic therapy that includes autologous HSCT. Squamous Cell Carcinoma of the Head and Neck (SCCHN) • patients with recurrent or metastatic squamous cell carcinoma of the head and neck with disease progression on or after a platinum-based therapy. Urothelial Carcinoma • patients with locally advanced or metastatic urothelial carcinoma • have disease progression during or following platinum-containing chemotherapy • have disease progression within 12 months of neoadjuvant or adjuvant treatment with platinum-containing chemotherapy. Colorectal Cancer • adult and pediatric (12 years and older) patients with microsatellite instability-high (MSI-H) or mismatch repair

		deficient (dMMR) metastatic colorectal cancer that has progressed following treatment with a fluoropyrimidine, oxaliplatin, and irinotecan, as a single agent or in combination with ipilimumab. Hepatocellular Carcinoma (HCC) • patients with hepatocellular carcinoma who have been previously treated with sorafenib, as a single agent or in combination with ipilimumab. Esophageal Squamous Cell Carcinoma (ESCC) • patients with unresectable advanced, recurrent or metastatic esophageal squamous cell carcinoma after prior fluoropyrimidine- and platinum-based chemotherapy. This indication is approved under accelerated approval based on overall response rate and duration of response. Continued approval for this indication may be contingent upon verification and description of clinical benefit in confirmatory trials.
Obiltoxaximab/ Anthim/ chimeric	Protective antigen of the Anthrax toxin	Adult and pediatric patients for treatment of inhalational anthrax due to B. anthracis in combination with appropriate antibacterial drugs and, for prophylaxis of inhalational anthrax when alternative therapies are not available or are not appropriate.
Obinutuzumab /Gazyva/ humanized	CD20	1.In combination with chlorambucil, for the treatment of patients with previously untreated chronic lymphocytic leukemia 2. In combination with bendamustine followed by GAZYVA monotherapy, for the treatment of patients with follicular lymphoma who relapsed after, or are refractory to, a rituximab-containing regimen. 3. In combination with chemotherapy followed by GAZYVA monotherapy in patients achieving at least a partial remission, for the treatment of adult patients with previously untreated stage II bulky, III or IV follicular lymphoma.
Ocrelizumab/ Ocrevus/ humanized	CD20	Relapsing or primary progressive forms of multiple sclerosis
Ofatumumab/ Arzerra/fully human	CD20	Chronic lymphocytic leukemia (CLL) refractory to fludarabine and alemtuzumab.
Olaratumab/ Lartruvo/fully human	PDGFR-α	In combination with doxorubicin, for the treatment of adult patients with soft tissue sarcoma (STS) with a histologic subtype for which an anthracycline-containing regimen is appropriate and which is not amenable to curative treatment with radiotherapy or surgery. This indication is approved under accelerated approval. Continued approval for this indication may be contingent upon verification and description of clinical benefit in the confirmatory trial

Omalizumab/ Xolair/ humanized	IgE	1.Moderate to severe persistent asthma in patients 6 years of age and older with a positive skin test or in vitro reactivity to a perennial aeroallergen and symptoms that are inadequately controlled with inhaled corticosteroids 2.Chronic idiopathic urticaria in adults and adolescents 12 years of age and older who remain symptomatic despite H1 antihistamine treatment
Palivizumab/ Synagis/ humanized	F protein of respiratory syncytial virus (RSV)	Prevention of serious lower respiratory tract disease caused by RSV in children at high risk of RSV disease. Notes 1. Safety and efficacy were established in children with bronchopulmonary dysplasia (BPD), infants with a history of premature birth (less than or equal to 35 weeks gestational age), and children with hemodynamically significant congenital heart disease (CHD). 2.The safety and efficacy of Synagis have not been established for treatment of RSV disease
Panitumumab/ Vectibix/ fully human	EGFR	As a single agent for the treatment of metastatic colorectal carcinoma with disease progression on or following fluoropyrimidine, oxaliplatin, and irinotecan chemotherapy regimens. Approval is based on progression-free survival; no data demonstrate an improvement in disease-related symptoms or increased survival with Vectibix. Notes 1. Retrospective subset analyses of metastatic colorectal cancer trials have not shown a treatment benefit for Vectibix in patients whose tumors had KRAS mutations in codon 12 or 13. 2.Use of Vectibix is not recommended for the treatment of colorectal cancer with these mutations
Pembrolizuma b/ Keytruda/ fully human	PD-1	Melanoma • for the treatment of patients with unresectable or metastatic melanoma. • for the adjuvant treatment of patients with melanoma with involvement of lymph node(s) following complete resection. Non-Small Cell Lung Cancer (NSCLC) • in combination with pemetrexed and platinum chemotherapy, as first-line treatment of patients with metastatic nonsquamous NSCLC, with no EGFR or ALK genomic tumor aberrations. • in combination with carboplatin and either paclitaxel or paclitaxel protein-bound, as first-line treatment of patients with metastatic squamous NSCLC. • as a single agent for the first-line treatment of patients with NSCLC expressing PD-L1 [Tumor Proportion Score (TPS) ≥1%] as determined by an FDA-approved test, with

		no EGFR or ALK genomic tumor aberrations, and is: o stage III where patients are not candidates for surgical resection or definitive chemoradiation, or o metastatic. • as a single agent for the treatment of patients with metastatic NSCLC whose tumors express PD-L1 (TPS ≥1%) as determined by an FDA-approved test, with disease progression on or after platinum-containing chemotherapy. Patients with EGFR or ALK genomic tumor aberrations should have disease progression on FDA-approved therapy for these aberrations prior to receiving KEYTRUDA. Small Cell Lung Cancer (SCLC) • for the treatment of patients with metastatic SCLC with disease progression on or after platinum-based chemotherapy and at least one other prior line of therapy. Head and Neck Squamous Cell Cancer (HNSCC) • in combination with platinum and FU for the first-line treatment of patients with metastatic or with unresectable, recurrent HNSCC. • as a single agent for the first-line treatment of patients with metastatic or with unresectable, recurrent HNSCC whose tumors express PD-L1 [Combined Positive Score (CPS) ≥1] as determined by an FDA-approved test. • as a single agent for the treatment of patients with recurrent or metastatic HNSCC with disease progression on or after platinum-containing chemotherapy. Classical Hodgkin Lymphoma (cHL) • for the treatment of adult patients with relapsed or refractory cHL. • for the treatment of pediatric patients with refractory cHL, or cHL that has relapsed after 2 or more lines of therapy. Primary Mediastinal Large B-Cell Lymphoma (PMBCL) • for the treatment of adult and pediatric patients with refractory PMBCL, or who have relapsed after 2 or more prior lines of therapy. • Limitations of Use: KEYTRUDA is not recommended for treatment of patients with PMBCL who require urgent cytoreductive therapy. Urothelial Carcinoma • for the treatment of patients with locally advanced or metastatic urothelial carcinoma who are not eligible for cisplatin-containing chemotherapy and whose tumors express PD-L1 [Combined Positive Score (CPS) ≥10] as

		determined by an FDA-approved test, or in patients who are not eligible for any platinum-containing chemotherapy regardless of PD-L1 status. • for the treatment of patients with locally advanced or metastatic urothelial carcinoma who have disease progression during or following platinum-containing chemotherapy or within 12 months of neoadjuvant or adjuvant treatment with platinum-containing chemotherapy. • for the treatment of patients with Bacillus Calmette-Guerin (BCG)-unresponsive, high-risk, non-muscle invasive bladder cancer (NMIBC) with carcinoma in situ (CIS) with or without papillary tumors who are ineligible for or have elected not to undergo cystectomy. Microsatellite Instability-High or Mismatch Repair Deficient Cancer • for the treatment of adult and pediatric patients with unresectable or metastatic, microsatellite instability-high (MSI-H) or mismatch repair deficient (dMMR) o solid tumors that have progressed following prior treatment and who have no satisfactory alternative treatment options,1 or o colorectal cancer that has progressed following treatment with a fluoropyrimidine, oxaliplatin, and irinotecan. • Limitations of Use: The safety and effectiveness of KEYTRUDA in pediatric patients with MSI-H central nervous system cancers have not been established. Microsatellite Instability-High or Mismatch Repair Deficient Colorectal Cancer (CRC) • for the first-line treatment of patients with unresectable or metastatic MSI-H or dMMR colorectal cancer (CRC). Gastric Cancer • for the treatment of patients with recurrent locally advanced or metastatic gastric or gastroesophageal junction adenocarcinoma whose tumors express PD-L1 [Combined Positive Score (CPS) ≥1] as determined by an FDA-approved test, with disease progression on or after 2 or more prior lines of therapy including fluoropyrimidine- and platinum-containing chemotherapy and if appropriate, HER2/neu-targeted therapy. Esophageal Cancer • for the treatment of patients with locally advanced or metastatic esophageal or gastroesophageal junction (GEJ) (tumors with epicenter 1 to 5 centimeters above the GEJ) carcinoma that is not amenable to surgical resection or definitive chemoradiation either:

		o in combination with platinum- and fluoropyrimidine-based chemotherapy, or o as a single agent after one or more prior lines of systemic therapy for patients with tumors of squamous cell histology that express PD-L1 (CPS ≥10) as determined by an FDA-approved test. Cervical Cancer • for the treatment of patients with recurrent or metastatic cervical cancer with disease progression on or after chemotherapy whose tumors express PD-L1 [Combined Positive Score (CPS) ≥1] as determined by an FDA-approved test. Hepatocellular Carcinoma (HCC) • for the treatment of patients with HCC who have been previously treated with sorafenib. Merkel Cell Carcinoma (MCC) • for the treatment of adult and pediatric patients with recurrent locally advanced or metastatic Merkel cell carcinoma. Renal Cell Carcinoma (RCC) • in combination with axitinib, for the first-line treatment of patients with advanced RCC. Endometrial Carcinoma • in combination with lenvatinib, for the treatment of patients with advanced endometrial carcinoma that is not MSI-H or dMMR, who have disease progression following prior systemic therapy and are not candidates for curative surgery or radiation. Tumor Mutational Burden-High (TMB-H) Cancer • for the treatment of adult and pediatric patients with unresectable or metastatic tumor mutational burden-high (TMB-H) ≥10 mutations/megabase (mut/Mb)] solid tumors, as determined by an FDA-approved test, that have progressed following prior treatment and who have no satisfactory alternative treatment options. • Limitations of Use: The safety and effectiveness of KEYTRUDA in pediatric patients with TMB-H central nervous system cancers have not been established. Cutaneous Squamous Cell Carcinoma (cSCC) • for the treatment of patients with recurrent or metastatic cutaneous squamous cell carcinoma that is not curable by surgery or radiation. Triple-Negative Breast Cancer (TNBC) • in combination with chemotherapy, for the treatment of patients with locally recurrent unresectable or metastatic

		TNBC whose tumors express PD-L1 [Combined Positive Score (CPS) ≥10] as determined by an FDA approved test. Adult Indications: additional dosing regimen of 400 mg every 6 Weeks • for use at an additional recommended dosage of 400 mg every 6 weeks for all approved adult indications. This indication is approved under accelerated approval based on tumor response rate and durability of response. Continued approval for this indication may be contingent upon verification and description of clinical benefit in the confirmatory trials.
Pertuzumab/ Perjeta/ humanized	HER2/neu	In combination with trastuzumab and docetaxel for the treatment of patients with HER2-positive metastatic breast cancer who have not received prior anti-HER2 therapy or chemotherapy for metastatic disease.
Polatuzumab vedotin/Polivy/ Humanized antibody-drug conjugate	CD79	In combination with bendamustine and a rituximab product for the treatment of adult patients with relapsed or refractory diffuse large B cell lymphoma, not otherwise specified, after at least two prior therapies
Ramucirumab/ Cyramza/ fully human	VEGFR2	1. As a single agent or in combination with paclitaxel, for treatment of advanced gastric or gastro-esophageal junction adenocarcinoma, with disease progression on or after prior fluoropyrimidine- or platinum-containing chemotherapy. 2. In combination with docetaxel, for treatment of metastatic non-small cell lung cancer with disease progression on or after platinum-based chemotherapy. Patients with EGFR or ALK genomic tumor aberrations should have disease progression on FDA-approved therapy for these aberrations prior to receiving CYRAMZA
Ranibizumab/ Lucentis/ humanized	VEGFR1, VEGFR2	1. Neovascular (wet) age-related macular degeneration (AMD) 2. Macular edema following retinal vein occlusion (RVO) 3. Diabetic macular edema (DME)
Raxibacumab/ fully human	Protective antigen of Bacillus anthracis[6]	Raxibacumab is indicated for the treatment of adult and pediatric patients with inhalational anthrax due to Bacillus anthracis in combination with appropriate antibacterial drugs, and for prophylaxis of inhalational anthrax when alternative therapies are not available or are not appropriate. Limitations of use: • The effectiveness of raxibacumab is based solely on efficacy studies in animal models of inhalational anthrax. • There have been no studies of raxibacumab in the pediatric population. Dosing in pediatric patients was derived using a population PK approach.

		• Raxibacumab does not cross the blood-brain barrier and does not prevent or treat meningitis. Raxibacumab should be used in combination with appropriate antibacterial drug
Reslizumab/ Cinqair/ humanized	IL-5	Add-on maintenance treatment of patients with severe asthma aged 18 years and older, and with an eosinophilic phenotype. Limitations of use: CINQAIR is not indicated for • treatment of other eosinophilic conditions • relief of acute bronchospasm or status asthmaticus
Rituximab/ Rituxan/ chimeric	CD20	1. Non-Hodgkin's lymphoma o Relapsed or refractory, low grade or follicular, CD20-positive B as a single agent. o Previously untreated follicular, CD20-positive, B cell in combination with first line chemotherapy and, in patients achieving a complete or partial response to RITUXAN in combination with chemotherapy, as single-agent maintenance therapy. o Non-progressing (including stable disease), low-grade, CD20 positive, B cell as a single agent after first-line cyclophosphamide, vincristine, and prednisone (CVP) chemotherapy. o Previously untreated diffuse large B cell, CD20-positive in combination with (cyclophosphamide, doxorubicin, vincristine, and prednisone) (CHOP) or other anthracycline-based chemotherapy regimens. 2. Chronic lymphocytic leukemia (CLL) o Previously untreated and previously treated CD20 positive CLL in combination with fludarabine and cyclophosphamide (FC). 3. Rheumatoid arthritis (RA) in combination with methotrexate in adult patients with moderately-to severely-active RA who have inadequate response to one or more TNF antagonist therapies 4. Granulomatosis with polyangiitis (GPA) (Wegener's granulomatosis) and microscopic polyangiitis (MPA) in adult patients in combination with glucocorticoids 5. Moderate to severe pemphigus vulgaris (PV) in adult patients
Rituximab and hyaluronidase/ chimeric co-formulated with hyaluronidase (a human endoglycos-idase)	CD20	1. Follicular lymphoma (FL) o Relapsed or refractory, follicular lymphoma as a single agent o Previously untreated follicular lymphoma in combination with first line chemotherapy and, in patients achieving a complete or partial response to rituximab in combination with chemotherapy, as single agent maintenance therapy

		o Non-progressing (including stable disease), follicular lymphoma as a single agent after first-line cyclophosphamide, vincristine, and prednisone (CVP) chemotherapy 2. Diffuse large B cell lymphoma (DLBCL) o Previously untreated diffuse large B cell lymphoma in combination with cyclophosphamide, doxorubicin, vincristine, prednisone (CHOP) or other anthracycline-based chemotherapy regimens 3. Chronic lymphocytic leukemia (CLL) o Previously untreated and previously treated CLL in combination with fludarabine and cyclophosphamide (FC) Limitations of use: • Initiate treatment with RITUXAN HYCELA only after patients have received at least one full d • RITUXAN HYCELA is not indicated for the treatment of non- conditions.
Sacituzumab govitecan-hziy/ TRODELVY Antibody-drug conjugate	Trop-2 Sacituzumab govitecan-hziy is a Trop-2-directed antibody-drug conjugate. Sacituzumab is a humanized antibody that recognizes Trop-2. The small molecule, SN-38, is a topoisomerase I inhibitor, which is covalently attached to the antibody by a linker. Pharmacology data suggest that sacituzumab govitecan-hziy binds to Trop-2-expressing cancer cells and is internalized with the subsequent release of SN-38 via hydrolysis of the linker. SN-38 interacts with topoisomerase I and prevents re-ligation of topoisomerase I-induced single	TRODELVY is a Trop-2-directed antibody and topoisomerase inhibitor conjugate indicated for the treatment of adult patients with metastatic triple-negative breast cancer (mTNBC) who have received at least two prior therapies for metastatic disease. This indication is approved under accelerated approval based on tumor response rate and duration of response. Continued approval for this indication may be contingent upon verification and description of clinical benefit in confirmatory trials

	strand breaks. The resulting DNA damage leads to apoptosis and cell death. Sacituzumab govitecan-hziy decreased tumor growth in mouse xenograft models of triple-negative breast cancer.	
Sarilumab/ Kevzara/ fully human	IL-6 receptor	Adult patients with moderately to severely active rheumatoid arthritis who have had an inadequate response or intolerance to one or more disease-modifying antirheumatic drugs
Satralizumab-mwge/ Enspryng Humanized	Satralizumab is a humanized monoclonal antibody targeted against human IL-6 receptors. It binds to soluble and membrane-bound IL-6 receptors and prevents the signaling cascade, and subsequent pro-inflammatory effects, associated with its binding to endogenous IL-6.	Treatment of neuromyelitis optica spectrum disorder (NMOSD) in adult patients who are anti-aquaporin-4 (AQP4)
Secukinumab/ Cosentryx/ fully human	IL-17A (also known as IL-17)	Moderate to severe plaque psoriasis in adult patients who are candidates for systemic therapy or phototherapy.
Siltuximab/ Sylvant/ chimeric	IL-6	Multicentric Castleman's disease (MCD) who are human immunodeficiency virus (HIV) negative and human herpesvirus-8 (HHV-8) negative.
Tafasitamab-cxix/ MONJUVI	CD19	MONJUVI is a CD19-directed cytolytic antibody indicated in combination with lenalidomide for the treatment of adult patients with relapsed or refractory diffuse large B cell lymphoma (DLBCL) not otherwise specified, including DLBCL arising from low grade lymphoma, and who are not eligible for autologous stem cell transplant (ASCT). Tafasitamab-cxix is an Fc-modified monoclonal antibody that binds to CD19 antigen expressed on the surface of pre-B and mature B lymphocytes and on several B cell malignancies, including diffuse large B cell lymphoma (DLBCL). Upon binding to CD19, tafasitamab-cxix mediates B cell lysis through apoptosis and immune

		effector mechanisms, including antibody-dependent cellular cytotoxicity (ADCC) and antibody-dependent cellular phagocytosis (ADCP). This indication is approved under accelerated approval based on overall response rate. Continued approval for this indication may be contingent upon verification and description of clinical benefit in a confirmatory trial(s)
Teprotumumab-trbw/ TEPEZZA	IGFR Teprotumumab-trbw's mechanism of action in patients with Thyroid Eye Disease has not been fully characterized. Teprotumumab-trbw binds to IGF-1R and blocks its activation and signaling	TEPEZZA is an insulin-like growth factor-1 receptor inhibitor indicated for the treatment of Thyroid Eye Disease
Tildrakizumab-asmn/Ilumya/ humanized	IL-23	Adults with moderate-to-severe plaque psoriasis who are candidates for systemic therapy or phototherapy
Tocilizumab/ Actrema/ humanized	IL-6 receptor	1. Rheumatoid arthritis (RA) • Adult patients with moderately to severely active rheumatoid arthritis who have had an inadequate response to one or more disease modifying anti-rheumatic drugs (DMARDs). 2.Giant cell arteritis (GCA) • Adult patients with giant cell arteritis. 3.Polyarticular juvenile idiopathic arthritis (PJIA) • Patients 2 years of age and older with active polyarticular juvenile idiopathic arthritis. 4.Systemic juvenile idiopathic arthritis (SJIA) • Patients 2 years of age and older with active systemic juvenile idiopathic arthritis. 5.Cytokine release syndrome (CRS) • Adults and pediatric patients 2 years of age and older with chimeric antigen receptor (CAR) T cell-induced severe or life-threatening cytokine release syndrome
Tratuzumab/ Herceptin/ humanized	HER2/neu	• HER2 overexpressing breast cancer •HER2-overexpressing metastatic gastric or gastroesophageal junction adenocarcinoma
Trastuzumab-dkst/Ogivri/ humanized biosimilar	HER2/neu	• HER2 overexpressing breast cancer •HER2-overexpressing metastatic gastric or gastroesophageal junction adenocarcinoma

Ustekinumab/ Stelara/ fully human	IL-12, IL-23	1. Adult patients with moderate to severe plaque psoriasis (Ps) who are candidates for phototherapy or systemic therapy. 2. Active psoriatic arthritis (PsA), alone or in combination with methotrexate. 3. Moderately to severely active Crohn's disease (CD) who have failed or were intolerant to treatment with immunomodulators or corticosteroids, but never failed a tumor necrosis factor (TNF) blocker or failed or were intolerant to treatment with one or more TNF blockers 4. Adolescent patients (12 years or older) with moderate to severe plaque psoriasis, who are candidates for phototherapy or systemic therapy
Vedolizumab/ Entyvio/ humanized	Binds to the α4β7 integrin and blocks the interaction of α4β7 integrin with mucosal addressin cell adhesion molecule-1 (MAdCAM-1) and inhibits the migration of memory T lymphocytes across the endothelium into inflamed gastro-intestinal parenchymal tissue	1. Adult ulcerative colitis (UC) Adult patients with moderately to severely active UC who have had an inadequate response with, lost response to, or were intolerant to a tumor necrosis factor (TNF) blocker or immunomodulator; or had an inadequate response with, were intolerant to, or demonstrated dependence on corticosteroids • inducing and maintaining clinical response • inducing and maintaining clinical remission • improving endoscopic appearance of the mucosa 2. Achieving corticosteroid-free remission adult Crohn's disease (CD) • Adult patients with moderately to severely active CD who have had an inadequate response with, lost response to, or were intolerant to a TNF blocker or immunomodulator; or had an inadequate response with, were intolerant to, or demonstrated dependence on corticosteroids • achieving clinical response • achieving clinical remission • achieving corticosteroid-free remission

[a]Hidradenitis suppuriva is long term skin disease characterized by the occurrence of inflamed and swollen lumps

One other FDA-approved mab, tositumomab (Bexxar) (anti-CD20), was discontinued in 2014 due to lack of demand

[1]Burrill Bernard Crohn (1884 – 1983) was an American gastroenterologist

[2]Friedrich Sigmund Merkel (1845-1919) was a German anatomist and histopathologist

[3]Thomas Hodgkin (1798 – 1866) was a British physician

[4]Albert Sézary (1880 – 1956) was a French dermatologist and syphilogist

[5] Benjamin Castleman (1906 – 1982) was an American physician and pathologist

Examples of other biological therapeutics approved by the FDA for non-malignant diseases and malignant diseases

- Janus kinase inhibitors – eg, tofacitinib in Crohn's disease, ruxolitinib for steroid-refractory acute graft-versus-host disease
- Bruton's tyrosine kinase inhibitor – eg, ibrutinib for chronic graft-versus-host disease
- Other human tyrosine kinase inhibitors – eg, imatinib for systemic mastocytosis
- Angiogenesis inhibitors – eg, aflibercept for diabetic retinopathy
- Small interfering RNA-based drugs- eg, onasemnogene abeparvovec-xioi (Zolgensma) for familial amyloid polyneuropathy

Enzyme replacement treatments – eg, cerliponase alfa (Brineura) for Batten disease

Enzyme inhibitors – eg, lanadelumab-flyo (Takhzyro) for hereditary angioedema

Anti-sense drugs - eg, fomivirsen for cytomegalovirus retinitis, mipomersen for homozygous familial hypercholesterolemia, eteplirsen for Duchenne muscular dystrophy, nusinersen for spinal muscular atrophy

Cell therapies – Umbilical cord blood stem cells: FDA-approved for over 80 diseases, both non-malignant and malignant.

Gene-modified cell therapies

As of December 2020, the FDA had approved three different chimeric antigen receptor (CAR) T cell therapeutic agents for B cell acute lymphoblastic leukemia and aggressive non-Hodgkin lymphomas.

Gene therapies – eg, onasemnogene abeparvovec-xioi (Zolgensma) to treat spinal muscular atrophy type 1 has been approved for therapeutic use by the FDA. Voretigene neparvovec-rzyl (Luxturna) to treat congenital retinal dystrophy has also been approved by the FDA.

Hedgehog pathway inhibitors – eg sonidegib and vismodegib. These agents are chemically synthesised and FDA-approved for the treatment of advanced cutaneous squamous cell carcinoma or advanced basal cell carcinoma of the skin.

M-TOR inhibitors – eg sirolimus, temsirolimus and everolimus which inhibit the kinase activity of m-TOR, and which are used as immune suppressive agents

A list of small molecule protein kinase inhibitors approved by the USA FDA for therapeutic use (as of December 2020) is shown in Table 2.

Table 2

Generic name/ trade name	**Target and mechanism of action**	**FDA-approved indication/s**
Abemaciclib/ Verzenio	Cyclin-dependent kinases 4 and 6 (CDK4 and CDK6). CDK4/6 inhibitor activity enforces G1 cell cycle arrest, and thus inhibits cellular proliferation	• In combination with an aromatase inhibitor as initial endocrine-based therapy for the treatment of postmenopausal women with hormone receptor (HR)-positive, human epidermal growth factor receptor 2 (HER2)-negative advanced or metastatic breast cancer. • in combination with fulvestrant for the treatment of women with hormone receptor (HR)-positive, human epidermal growth factor receptor 2 (HER2)-negative advanced or metastatic breast cancer with disease progression following endocrine therapy. • as monotherapy for the treatment of adult patients with HR positive, HER2-negative advanced or metastatic breast cancer with disease progression following endocrine therapy and prior chemotherapy in the metastatic setting.
Acalabrutinib/ Calquence	Bruton's tyrosine kinase[1]. (BTK). BTK is a signalling molecule of the B cell antigen receptor (BCR)	1. Mantle cell lymphoma (MCL) who have received at least one prior therapy. This indication is

	and cytokine receptor pathways	approved under accelerated approval based on overall response rate. Continued approval for this indication may be contingent upon verification and description of clinical benefit in confirmatory trials 2. Chronic lymphocytic leukemia (CLL) or small lymphocytic lymphoma (SLL)
Afatinib/ Golotrif	ErbB (derived avian erythroblastosis oncogeneB). Signalling through the ErbB1/2/4 family of receptors promotes cell proliferation and opposes apoptosis. (ErbB is also known as, HER-2, HER-2/neu, HER2, NEU, CD340). Afatinib covalently binds to the kinase domains of EGFR (ErbB1), HER2 (ErbB2), and HER4 (ErbB4) and irreversibly inhibits tyrosine kinase autophosphorylation, resulting in downregulation of ErbB signalling.	1. First-line treatment of patients with metastatic non-small cell lung cancer (NSCLC) whose tumors have non-resistant epidermal growth factor receptor (EGFR) mutations 2. Treatment of patients with metastatic, squamous NSCLC progressing after platinum-based chemotherapy
Alectinib/ Alecensa	ALK, RET. Alectinib is a tyrosine kinase inhibitor that targets ALK and RET. In non-clinical studies, alectinib inhibited ALK phosphorylation and ALK-mediated activation of the downstream signalling proteins STAT3 and AKT, and decreased tumor cell viability in multiple cell lines harboring ALK fusions, amplifications, or activating mutations.	Anaplastic lymphoma kinase (ALK)-positive metastatic non-small cell lung cancer (NSCLC)
Avapritinib/AYVAKIT	PDGFRA and PDGFRA D842 mutants Avapritinib is a tyrosine kinase inhibitor that targets PDGFRA and PDGFRA D842 mutants as well as multiple KIT exon 11, 11/17 and 17 mutants with half maximal inhibitory concentrations (IC50s) less than 25 nM. Certain mutations in PDGFRA and KIT can result in the autophosphorylation and constitutive activation of these receptors which can contribute to tumor cell proliferation. Other potential targets for avapritinib include wild type KIT, PDGFRB, and CSFR1. In in vitro	AYVAKIT is a kinase inhibitor indicated for the treatment of adults with unresectable or metastatic gastrointestinal stromal tumor (GIST) harboring a platelet-derived growth factor receptor alpha (PDGFRA) exon 18 mutation, including PDGFRA D842V mutations.

	cellular assays, avapritinib inhibited the autophosphorylation of KIT D816V and PDGFRA D842V, mutants associated with resistance to approved kinase inhibitors, with IC50 of 4 nM and 30 nM, respectively. Avapritinib also had anti-tumor activity in mice implanted with an imatinib-resistant patientderived xenograft model of human GIST with activating KIT exon 11/17 mutations.	
Axitinib/Inlyta	Vascular endothelial growth factor receptors (VEGFR) 1/2/3. Axitinib has been shown to inhibit receptor tyrosine kinases including vascular endothelial growth factor receptors VEGFR-1, VEGFR-2, and VEGFR-3	Advanced renal cell carcinoma after failure of one prior systemic therapy
Baricitinib/ Olumiant	JAK1/2. Janus kinases phosphorylate activated cytokine receptors. These phosphorylated receptors in turn recruit STAT transcrip-tion factors which modulate gene transcription	Adult patients with moderately to severely active rheumatoid arthritis who have had an inadequate response to one or more TNF antagonist therapies
Binimetinib/ Mektovi	MEK1/2. MEK inhibitors inhibit the mitogen-activated protein kinase kinase enzymes MEK1and/or MEK2. They can be used to affect the MAPK/ERK pathway which is often overactive in some cancers	In combination with encorafenib, for the treatment of patients with unresectable or metastatic melanoma with a BRAF V600E or V600K mutation, as detected by an FDA-approved test.
Bosutinib/ Bosulif	BCR-ABL Bosutinib inhibits the BCR-ABL kinase that promotes CML	Treatment of adult patients with chronic, accelerated, or blast phase Ph+ chronic myelogenous leukemia (CML) with resistance or intolerance to prior therapy
Brigatinib/ Alunbrig	ALK. Brigatinib is a tyrosine kinase inhibitor with in vitro activity at clinically achievable concentrations against multiple kinases including ALK, ROS1, insulin-like growth factor-1 receptor (IGF-1R), and FLT-3 as well as EGFR deletion and point mutations. Brigatinib inhibited autophosphorylation of ALK and ALK-mediated phosphorylation of the downstream signalling proteins STAT3, AKT, ERK1/2, and S6 in in vitro and in vivo assays.	Patients with anaplastic lymphoma kinase (ALK)-positive metastatic non-small cell lung cancer (NSCLC) who have progressed on or are intolerant to crizotinib. This indication is approved under accelerated approval based on tumor response rate and duration of response. Continued approval for this indication may be contingent upon verification and description of clinical benefit in a confirmatory trial

Cabozantinib/ Cabometyx	RET, VEGFR2. Cabozantinib inhibits the tyrosine kinase activity of RET, MET, VEGFR-1, -2 and -3, KIT, TRKB, FLT-3, AXL, ROS1, TYRO3, MER, and TIE-2. These receptor tyrosine kinases are involved in both normal cellular function and pathologic processes such as oncogenesis, metastasis, tumor angiogenesis, drug resistance, and maintenance of the tumor microenvironment.	1.Patients with advanced renal cell carcinoma (RCC) 2. Patients with hepatocellular carcinoma (HCC) who have been previously treated with sorafenib
Cabozantinib/ Cometriq	RET, VEGFR2	Patients with progressive, metastatic medullary thyroid cancer (MTC)
Capmatinib/ TABRECTATM	MET Capmatinib is a kinase inhibitor that targets MET, including the mutant variant produced by exon 14 skipping. MET exon 14 skipping results in a protein with a missing regulatory domain that reduces its negative regulation leading to increased downstream MET signaling. Capmatinib inhibited cancer cell growth driven by a mutant MET variant lacking exon 14 at clinically achievable concentrations and demonstrated anti-tumor activity in murine tumor xenograft models derived from human lung tumors with either a mutation leading to MET exon 14 skipping or MET amplification. Capmatinib inhibited the phosphorylation of MET triggered by binding of hepatocyte growth factor or by MET amplification, as well as METmediated phosphorylation of downstream signaling proteins and proliferation and survival of MET-dependent cancer cells.	TABRECTA is a kinase inhibitor indicated for the treatment of adult patients with metastatic non-small cell lung cancer (NSCLC) whose tumors have a mutation that leads to mesenchymal-epithelial transition (MET) exon 14 skipping as detected by an FDA-approved test. This indication is approved under accelerated approval based on overall response rate and duration of response. Continued approval for this indication may be contingent upon verification and description of clinical benefit in confirmatory trial(s).
Ceritinib/ Zykadia	ALK. Targets of ceritinib inhibition identified in either biochemical or cellular assays at clinically relevant concentrations include ALK, insulin-like growth factor 1 receptor (IGF-1R), insulin receptor (InsR), and ROS1. Among these, ceritinib is most active against ALK. Ceritinib inhibited autophosphorylation of ALK, ALK-mediated phosphorylation of the downstream signalling protein STAT3, and proliferation of ALK-dependent cancer cells in in vitro and	Patients with metastatic non-small cell lung cancer (NSCLC) whose tumors are anaplastic lymphoma kinase (ALK)-positive

	in vivo assays.	
Cobimetinib/ Cotellic	MEK1/2. Cobimetinib is a reversible inhibitor of mitogen-activated protein kinase (MAPK)/extracellular signal regulated kinase 1 (MEK1) and MEK2. MEK proteins are upstream regulators of the extracellular signal related kinase (ERK) pathway, which promotes cellular proliferation. BRAF V600E and K mutations result in constitutive activation of the BRAF pathway which includes MEK1 and MEK2.	Unresectable or metastatic melanoma with a BRAF V600E or V600K mutation, in combination with vemurafenib
Crizotinib/ Xalkori	ALK, ROS1. Crizotinib is an inhibitor of receptor tyrosine kinases including ALK, Hepatocyte growth factor receptor (HGFR, c-Met), ROS1 (c-ros), and Recepteur d'Origine Nantais (RON). Translocations can affect the ALK gene resulting in the expression of oncogenic fusion proteins. The formation of ALK fusion proteins results in activation and dysregulation of the gene's expression and signalling which can contribute to increased cell proliferation and survival in tumors expressing these proteins.	Patients with metastatic non-small cell lung cancer (NSCLC) whose tumors are anaplastic lymphoma kinase (ALK) or ROS1-positive
Dabrafenib/ Tafinlar	B-RAF. Dabrafenib is an inhibitor of some mutated forms of BRAF kinases with in vitro IC50 values of 0.65, 0.5, and 1.84 nM for BRAF V600E, BRAF V600K, and BRAF V600D enzymes, respectively. Dabrafenib also inhibits wild-type BRAF and CRAF kinases with IC50 values of 3.2 and 5.0 nM, respectively, and other kinases such as SIK1, NEK11, and LIMK1 at higher concentrations. Some mutations in the BRAF gene, including those that result in BRAF V600E, can result in constitutively activated BRAF kinases that may stimulate tumor cell growth.	TAFINLAR is a kinase inhibitor indicated as a single agent for the treatment of patients with unresectable or metastatic melanoma with BRAF V600E mutation as detected by an FDA-approved test. • TAFINLAR in combination with trametinib is indicated for the treatment of patients with unresectable or metastatic melanoma with BRAF V600E or V600K mutations as detected by an FDA-approved test. The use in combination is based on the demonstration of durable response rate. Improvement in disease-related symptoms or overall survival has not been demonstrated for TAFINLAR in combination with trametinib. Limitation of Use: TAFINLAR is not indicated for treatment of patients with wild-type BRAF melanoma.

Dacomitinib/ Vizimpro	EGFR. Dacomitinib is an irreversible inhibitor of the kinase activity of the human epidermal growth factor receptor (EGFR) family (EGFR/HER1, HER2, and HER4) and certain EGFR activating mutations (exon 19 deletion or the exon 21 L858R substitution mutation).	First-line treatment of patients with metastatic non-small cell lung cancer (NSCLC) with epidermal growth factor receptor (EGFR) exon 19 deletion or exon 21 L858R substitution mutations
Dasatinib/ Sprycell	BCR-ABL. Dasatinib, at nanomolar concentrations, inhibits the following kinases: BCR-ABL, SRC family (SRC, LCK, YES, FYN), c-KIT, EPHA2, and PDGFR-β. Based on modeling studies, dasatinib is predicted to bind to multiple conformations of the ABL kinase.	1. Newly diagnosed adults with Philadelphia chromosome-positive (Ph+) chronic myeloid leukemia (CML) in chronic phase. The trial is ongoing and further data will be required to determine long-term outcome. 2. Adults with chronic, accelerated, or myeloid or lymphoid blast phase Ph+ CML with resistance or intolerance to prior therapy including imatinib. 3. Adults with Philadelphia chromosome-positive acute lymphoblastic leukemia (Ph+ ALL) with resistance or intolerance to prior therapy
Encorafenib/Braftovi	B-RAF. Encorafenib is a kinase inhibitor that targets BRAF V600E, as well as wild-type BRAF and CRAF in in vitro cell-free assays with IC50 values of 0.35, 0.47, and 0.3 nM, respectively. Mutations in the BRAF gene, such as BRAF V600E, can result in constitutively activated BRAF kinases that may stimulate tumor cell growth. Encorafenib was also able to bind to other kinases in vitro including JNK1, JNK2, JNK3, LIMK1, LIMK2, MEK4, and STK36 and substantially reduce ligand binding to these kinases at clinically achievable concentrations ($\leq$ 0.9 μM).	BRAFTOVI is a kinase inhibitor indicated: • in combination with binimetinib, for the treatment of patients with unresectable or metastatic melanoma with a BRAF V600E or V600K mutation, as detected by an FDA-approved test. • in combination with cetuximab, for the treatment of adult patients with metastatic colorectal cancer (CRC) with a BRAF V600E mutation, as detected by an FDA-approved test, after prior therapy. Limitations of Use: BRAFTOVI is not indicated for treatment of patients with wild-type BRAF melanoma or wild-type BRAF CRC.
Entrectinib/ Rozlytrek	TRKA/B/C, ROS1, ALK. Entrectinib is an inhibitor of the tropomyosin receptor tyrosine kinases (TRK) TRKA, TRKB, and TRKC (encoded by the neurotrophic tyrosine receptor kinase [NTRK] genes NTRK1, NTRK2, and NTRK3,	• Adult patients with metastatic non-small cell lung cancer (NSCLC) whose tumors are ROS1-positive • Adult and pediatric patients 12 years of age and older with solid

	respectively), proto-oncogene tyrosine-protein kinase ROS1 (ROS1), and anaplastic lymphoma kinase (ALK). Fusion proteins that include TRK, ROS1, or ALK kinase domains can drive tumorigenic potential through hyperactivation of downstream signalling pathways leading to unconstrained cell proliferation.	tumors that: o have a neurotrophic tyrosine receptor kinase (NTRK) gene fusion without a known acquired resistance mutation o are metastatic or where surgical resection is likely to result in severe morbidity o have progressed following treatment or have no satisfactory alternative therapy. This indication is approved under accelerated approval based on tumor response rate and durability of response. Continued approval for this indication may be contingent upon verification and description of clinical benefit in the confirmatory trials.
Erdafitinib/ Balversa	FGFR1/2/3/4. Erdafitinib is a kinase inhibitor that binds to and inhibits enzymatic activity of FGFR1, FGFR2, FGFR3 and FGFR4 based on in vitro data. Erdafitinib also binds to RET, CSF1R, PDGFRA, PDGFRB, FLT4, KIT, and VEGFR2. Erdafitinib inhibited FGFR phosphorylation and signalling and decreased cell viability in cell lines expressing FGFR genetic alterations, including point mutations, amplifications, and fusions. Erdafitinib demonstrated antitumor activity in FGFR-expressing cell lines and xenograft models derived from tumor types, including bladder cancer.	Treatment of adult patients with locally advanced or metastatic urothelial carcinoma that has • susceptible FGFR3 or FGFR2 genetic alterations and • progressed during or following at least one line of prior platinum-containing chemotherapy including within 12 months of neoadjuvant or adjuvant platinum-containing chemotherapy. This indication is approved under accelerated approval based on tumor response rate. Continued approval for this indication may be contingent upon verification and description of clinical benefit in confirmatory trials
Erlotinib/ Tarceva	EGFR. The mechanism of the clinical antitumor action of erlotinib is not fully characterized. Erlotinib inhibits the intracellular phosphorylation of tyrosine kinase associated with the epidermal growth factor receptor (EGFR). Specificity of inhibition with regard to other tyrosine kinase receptors has not been fully characterized. EGFR is expressed on the cell surface of normal cells and cancer cells.	1. Maintenance treatment of patients with locally advanced or metastatic non-small cell lung cancer (NSCLC) whose disease has not progressed after four cycles of platinum-based first-line chemotherapy. 2.Treatment of locally advanced or metastatic non-small cell lung cancer after failure of at least one prior chemotherapy regimen. 3.First-line treatment of patients with locally advanced, unresectable or metastatic pancreatic cancer, in combination

		with gemcitabine
Fedratinib/ Inrebic	JAK2, FLT3. Fedratinib is an oral kinase inhibitor with activity against wild type and mutationally activated Janus Associated Kinase 2 (JAK2) and FMS-like tyrosine kinase 3 (FLT3). Fedratinib is a JAK2-selective inhibitor with higher inhibitory activity for JAK2 over family members JAK1, JAK3 and TYK2. Abnormal activation of JAK2 is associated with myeloproliferative neoplasms (MPNs), including myelofibrosis and polycythemia vera	Treatment of adult patients with intermediate-2 or high-risk primary or secondary (post-polycythemia vera or post-essential thrombocythemia) myelofibrosis (MF)
Fostamatinib/ Tavalisse	SYK. Fostamatinib is a tyrosine kinase inhibitor with demonstrated activity against spleen tyrosine kinase (SYK). The major metabolite of fostamatinib, R406, inhibits signal transduction of Fc-activating receptors and B cell receptor. The fostamatinib metabolite R406 reduces antibody-mediated destruction of platelets.	Treatment of thrombocytopenia in adult patients with chronic immune thrombocytopenia (ITP) who have had an insufficient response to a previous treatment.
Gefitinib/ Iressa	EGFR. The epidermal growth factor receptor (EGFR) is expressed on the cell surface of both normal and cancer cells and plays a role in the processes of cell growth and proliferation. Some EGFR activating mutations (exon 19 deletion or exon 21 point mutation L858R) within NSCLC cells have been identified as contributing to the promotion of tumor cell growth, blocking of apoptosis, increasing the production of angiogenic factors and facilitating the processes of metastasis. Gefitinib reversibly inhibits the kinase activity of wild-type and certain activating mutations of EGFR, preventing autophosphorylation of tyrosine residues associated with the receptor, thereby inhibiting further downstream signalling and blocking EGFR-dependent proliferation. Gefitinib binding affinity for EGFR exon 19 deletion or exon 21 point mutation L858R mutations is higher than its affinity for the wild-type EGFR. Gefitinib also inhibits IGF and PDGF-mediated signalling at clinically relevant concentrations; inhibition of other tyrosine kinase	First-line treatment of patients with metastatic non-small cell lung cancer (NSCLC) whose tumors have epidermal growth factor receptor (EGFR) exon 19 deletions or exon 21 (L858R) substitution mutations. Limitation of use: the safety and efficacy of IRESSA have not been established in patients whose tumors have EGFR mutations other than exon 19 deletions or exon 21 (L858R) substitution mutations

	receptors has not been fully characterized.	
Gilteritinib/ Xospata	Flt3. Gilteritinib is a small molecule that inhibits multiple receptor tyrosine kinases, including FMS-like tyrosine kinase 3 (FLT3). Gilteritinib demonstrated the ability to inhibit FLT3 receptor signalling and proliferation in cells exogenously expressing FLT3 including FLT3-ITD, tyrosine kinase domain mutations (TKD) FLT3-D835Y and FLT3-ITD-D835, and it induced apoptosis in leukemic cells expressing FLT3-ITD.	Treatment of adult patients who have relapsed or refractory acute myeloid leukemia (AML) with a FLT3 mutation
Ibrutinib/ Imbruvica	BTK. Ibrutinib is a small-molecule inhibitor of BTK. Ibrutinib forms a covalent bond with a cysteine residue in the BTK active site, leading to inhibition of BTK enzymatic activity. BTK is a signalling molecule of the B cell antigen receptor (BCR) and cytokine receptor pathways. BTK's role in signalling through the B cell surface receptors results in activation of pathways necessary for B cell trafficking, chemotaxis, and adhesion. Non-clinical studies show that ibrutinib inhibits B cell proliferation and survival in vivo as well as cell migration and substrate adhesion in vitro.	Treatment of adult patients with: 1. Mantle cell lymphoma (MCL) who have received at least one prior therapy. Accelerated approval was granted for this indication based on overall response rate. Continued approval for this indication may be contingent upon verification and description of clinical benefit in a confirmatory trial. 2. Chronic lymphocytic leukemia (CLL)/Small lymphocytic lymphoma (SLL) Chronic lymphocytic leukemia (CLL)/Small lymphocytic lymphoma (SLL) with 17p deletion 3. Waldenström's macroglobulinemia (WM) 4. Marginal zone lymphoma (MZL) who require systemic therapy and have received at least one prior anti-CD20-based therapy. Accelerated approval was granted for this indication based on overall response rate. Continued approval for this indication may be contingent upon verification and description of clinical benefit in a confirmatory trial. 5. Chronic graft-versus-host disease (cGVHD) after failure of one or more lines of systemic therapy
Imatinib/ Gleevec	Imatinib is tyrosine kinase specific for the TK domain in abl (the Abelson proto-oncogene), c-kit and PDGF-R (platelet-derived growth	1. Newly diagnosed adult and pediatric patients with Philadelphia chromosome positive chronic myeloid leukemia (Ph+

	factor receptor.	CML) in chronic phase 2. Patients with Philadelphia chromosome positive chronic myeloid leukemia (Ph+ CML) in blast crisis (BC), accelerated phase (AP), or in chronic phase (CP) after failure of interferon-alpha therapy 3. Adult patients with relapsed or refractory Philadelphia chromosome positive acute lymphoblastic leukemia (Ph+ ALL) 4. Pediatric patients with newly diagnosed Philadelphia chromosome positive acute lymphoblastic leukemia (Ph+ ALL) in combination with chemotherapy 5. Adult patients with myelodysplastic/myeloproliferative diseases (MDS/MPD) associated with platelet-derived growth factor receptor (PDGFR) gene re-arrangements 6. Adult patients with aggressive systemic mastocytosis (ASM) without the D816V c-Kit mutation or with c-Kit mutational status unknown 7. Adult patients with hypereosinophilic syndrome (HES) and/or chronic eosinophilic leukemia (CEL) who have the FIP1L1-PDGFR-α fusion kinase and for patients with HES and/or CEL who are FIP1L1 PDGFR-α fusion kinase negative or unknown 8. Adult patients with unresectable, recurrent and/or metastatic dermatofibrosarcoma protuberans (DFSP) 9. Patients with kit (CD117) positive unresectable and/or metastatic gastrointestinal stromal tumors (GIST) 10. Adjuvant treatment of adult patients following resection of kit (CD117) positive GIST
Lapatinib/ Tykerb	EGFR, ErbB2/HER2. Lapatinib is a 4-anilinoquinazoline kinase inhibitor of the intracellular tyrosine kinase domains of both	TYKERB, a kinase inhibitor, is indicated in combination with: • capecitabine, for the treatment of patients with advanced or

	Epidermal Growth Factor Receptor (EGFR [ErbB1]) and of Human Epidermal Receptor Type 2 (HER2 [ErbB2]). Lapatinib inhibits ErbB-driven tumor cell growth in vitro and in various animal models.	metastatic breast cancer whose tumors overexpress HER2 and who have received prior therapy including an anthracycline, a taxane, and trastuzumab. • letrozole for the treatment of postmenopausal women with hormone receptor positive metastatic breast cancer that overexpresses the HER2 receptor for whom hormonal therapy is indicated. TYKERB in combination with an aromatase inhibitor has not been compared to a trastuzumab-containing chemotherapy regimen for the treatment of metastatic breast cancer
Larotrectinib/ Vitrakvi	TRKA/B/C. Larotrectinib is an inhibitor of the tropomyosin receptor kinases (TRK), TRKA, TRKB, and TRKC. In a broad panel of purified enzyme assays, larotrectinib inhibited TRKA, TRKB, and TRKC. TRKA, B, and C are encoded by the genes NTRK1, NTRK2, and NTRK3. Chromosomal rearrangements involving in-frame fusions of these genes with various partners can result in constitutively-activated chimeric TRK fusion proteins that can act as an oncogenic driver, promoting cell proliferation and survival in tumor cell lines.	Treatment of adult and pediatric patients with solid tumors that • have a neurotrophic receptor tyrosine kinase (NTRK) gene fusion without a known acquired resistance mutation • are metastatic or where surgical resection is likely to result in severe morbidity, and • have no satisfactory alternative treatments or that have progressed following treatment. This indication is approved under accelerated approval based on overall response rate and duration of response. Continued approval for this indication may be contingent upon verification and description of clinical benefit in confirmatory trials.
Lenvatinib/ Lenvima	VEGFR, FGFR, RET, PDGFR, KIT. Lenvatinib is a kinase inhibitor that inhibits the kinase activities of vascular endothelial growth factor (VEGF) receptors VEGFR1 (FLT1), VEGFR2 (KDR), and VEGFR3 (FLT4). Lenvatinib inhibits other kinases that have been implicated in pathogenic angiogenesis, tumor growth, and cancer progression in addition to their normal cellular functions, including fibroblast growth factor (FGF) receptors FGFR1, 2, 3, and 4; platelet derived growth factor receptor alpha (PDGFRα), KIT, and RET. Lenvatinib also exhibited	Treatment of patients with 1. Locally recurrent or metastatic, progressive, radioactive iodine-refractory differentiated thyroid cancer (DTC). 2. In combination with everolimus, for the treatment of patients with advanced renal cell carcinoma (RCC) following one prior antiangiogenic therapy. 3. For the first-line treatment of patients with unresectable hepatocellular carcinoma (HCC)

	antiproliferative activity in hepatocellular carcinoma cell lines dependent on activated FGFR signalling with a concurrent inhibition of FGF-receptor substrate 2α (FRS2α) phosphorylation. The combination of lenvatinib and everolimus showed increased antiangiogenic and antitumor activity as demonstrated by decreases in human endothelial cell proliferation, tube formation, and VEGF signalling in vitro, and by decreases in tumor volume in mouse xenograft models of human renal cell cancer that were greater than those with either drug alone.	
Lonafarnib	Lonafarnib inhibits farnesyltransferase to prevent farnesylation and subsequent accumulation of progerin and progerin-like proteins in the inner nuclear membrane.	ZOKINVY is a farnesyltransferase inhibitor indicated in patients 12 months of age and older with a body surface area of 0.39 m^2 and above • To reduce risk of mortality in Hutchinson-Gilford Progeria Syndrome • For treatment of processing-deficient Progeroid Laminopathies with either: o Heterozygous LMNA mutation with progerin-like protein accumulation o Homozygous or compound heterozygous ZMPSTE24 mutations
Lorlatinib/ Lorbrena	ALK, ROS1 and others. Lorlatinib is a kinase inhibitor with in vitro activity against ALK and ROS1 as well as TYK1, FER, FPS, TRKA, TRKB, TRKC, FAK, FAK2, and ACK. Lorlatinib demonstrated in vitro activity against multiple mutant forms of the ALK enzyme, including some mutations detected in tumors at the time of disease progression on crizotinib and other ALK inhibitors.	Treatment of patients with anaplastic lymphoma kinase (ALK)-positive metastatic non-small cell lung cancer (NSCLC) whose disease has progressed on • crizotinib and at least one other ALK inhibitor for metastatic disease • or on alectinib as the first ALK inhibitor therapy for metastatic disease • or on ceritinib as the first ALK inhibitor therapy for metastatic disease. This indication is approved under accelerated approval based on tumor response rate and duration of response. Continued approval for this indication may be

		contingent upon verification and description of clinical benefit in a confirmatory trial.
Midostaurin/ Rydapt	Flt3. Midostaurin is a small molecule that inhibits multiple receptor tyrosine kinases. In vitro biochemical or cellular assays have shown that midostaurin or its major human active metabolites CGP62221 and CGP52421 inhibit the activity of wild type FLT3, FLT3 mutant kinases (ITD and TKD), KIT (wild type and D816V mutant), PDGFRα/β, VEGFR2, as well as members of the serine/threonine kinase PKC (protein kinase C) family.	Treatment of adult patients with: newly diagnosed acute myeloid leukemia (AML) that is FLT3 mutation-positive in combination with standard cytarabine and daunorubicin induction and cytarabine consolidation. Limitations of use: RYDAPT is not indicated as a single-agent induction therapy for the treatment of patients with AML, aggressive systemic mastocytosis (ASM), systemic mastocytosis with associated hematological neoplasm (SM-AHN), or mast cell leukemia (MCL).
Neratinib/ Nerlynx	ErbB2/HER2. A kinase inhibitor that irreversibly binds to Epidermal Growth Factor Receptor (EGFR), Human Epidermal Growth Factor Receptor 2 (HER2), and HER4. In vitro, neratinib reduces EGFR and HER2 autophosphorylation, downstream MAPK and AKT signalling pathways, and showed antitumor activity in EGFR and/or HER2 expressing carcinoma cell lines. Neratinib human metabolites M3, M6, M7 and M11 inhibited the activity of EGFR, HER2 and HER4 in vitro. In vivo, oral administration of neratinib inhibited tumor growth in mouse xenograft models with tumor cell lines expressing HER2 and EGFR.	NERLYNX is a kinase inhibitor indicated: • As a single agent, for the extended adjuvant treatment of adult patients with early stage HER2-positive breast cancer, to follow adjuvant trastuzumabbased therapy. • In combination with capecitabine, for the treatment of adult patients with advanced or metastatic HER2-positive breast cancer who have received two or more prior anti-HER2 based regimens in the metastatic setting.
Netarsudil/ Rhopressa	ROCK1/2 (Rho associated coiled-coil containing protein kinase 1) Netarsudil is a rho kinase inhibitor, which is believed to reduce intra-ocular pressure (IOP) by increasing the outflow of aqueous humor through the trabecular meshwork route. The exact mechanism is unknown.	RHOPRESSA® (netarsudil ophthalmic solution) 0.02% is a Rho kinase inhibitor indicated for the reduction of elevated intraocular pressure in patients with open-angle glaucoma or ocular hypertension
Nilotinib/ Tasigna	BCR-ABL. Nilotinib is an inhibitor of the BCR-ABL kinase.	1. Treatment of newly diagnosed adult patients with Philadelphia chromosome positive chronic myeloid leukemia (Ph+ CML) in chronic phase. 2. Treatment of chronic phase (CP) and accelerated phase (AP)

		Ph+ CML in adult patients resistant to or intolerant to prior therapy that included imatinib.
Nintedanib/ Vargatef	Multiple kinases. Nintedanib is a small molecule that inhibits multiple receptor tyrosine kinases (RTKs) and non-receptor tyrosine kinases (nRTKs). Nintedanib inhibits the following RTKs: platelet-derived growth factor receptor (PDGFR) α and β, fibroblast growth factor receptor (FGFR) 1-3, vascular endothelial growth factor receptor (VEGFR) 1-3, and Fms-like tyrosine kinase-3 (FLT3). Among them, FGFR, PDGFR, and VEGFR have been implicated in IPF pathogenesis. Nintedanib binds competitively to the adenosine triphosphate (ATP) binding pocket of these receptors and blocks the intracellular signalling which is crucial for the proliferation, migration, and transformation of fibroblasts representing essential mechanisms of the IPF pathology.	The treatment of idiopathic pulmonary fibrosis (IPF).
Osimertinib/ Tagrisso	EGFR Osimertinib is a kinase inhibitor of the epidermal growth factor receptor (EGFR), which binds irreversibly to certain mutant forms of EGFR (T790M, L858R, and exon 19 deletion) at approximately 9- fold lower concentrations than wild-type. In vitro, osimertinib also inhibited the activity of HER2, HER3, HER4, ACK1, and BLK at clinically relevant concentrations. In cultured cells and animal tumor implantation models, osimertinib exhibited anti-tumor activity against NSCLC lines harboring EGFR-mutations (T790M/L858R, L858R, T790M/exon 19 deletion, and exon 19 deletion) and, to a lesser extent, wild-type EGFR amplifications	1. The first-line treatment of patients with metastatic NSCLC whose tumors have epidermal growth factor receptor (EGFR) exon 19 deletions or exon 21 L858R mutations 2. The treatment of patients with metastatic EGFR T790M mutation-positive NSCLC whose disease has progressed on or after EGFR TKI therapy
Palbociclib/ Ibrance	CDK4/6	IBRANCE is a kinase inhibitor indicated for the treatment of adult patients with hormone receptor (HR)-positive, human epidermal growth factor receptor 2 (HER2)-negative advanced or metastatic breast cancer in combination with: • an aromatase inhibitor as initial endocrine-based therapy in postmenopausal women or in

		men; or • fulvestrant in patients with disease progression following endocrine therapy.
Pazopanib/ Votrient	VEGFR1/2/3 Pazopanib is a multi-tyrosine kinase inhibitor of vascular endothelial growth factor receptor (VEGFR)-1, VEGFR-2, VEGFR-3, platelet-derived growth factor receptor (PDGFR)-α and -β, fibroblast growth factor receptor (FGFR) -1 and -3, cytokine receptor (Kit), interleukin-2, receptor inducible T cell kinase (Itk), leukocyte-specific protein tyrosine kinase (Lck), and transmembrane glycoprotein receptor tyrosine kinase (c-fms). In vitro, pazopanib inhibited ligand-induced autophosphorylation of VEGFR-2, Kit and PDGFR-β receptors. In vivo, pazopanib inhibited VEGF-induced VEGFR-2 phosphorylation in mouse lungs, angiogenesis in a mouse model, and the growth of some human tumor xenografts in mice.	The treatment of patients with: 1. Advanced renal cell carcinoma 2. Advanced soft tissue sarcoma who have received prior chemotherapy. Limitations of use: the efficacy of VOTRIENT for the treatment of patients with adipocytic soft tissue sarcoma or gastrointestinal stromal tumors has not been demonstrated.
Pemigatinib/ PEMAZYRE™	FGFR2 Pemigatinib is a small molecule kinase inhibitor that targets FGFR1, 2 and 3 with IC50 values of less than 2 nM. Pemigatinib also inhibited FGFR4 in vitro at a concentration approximately 100 times higher than those that inhibit FGFR1, 2, and 3. Pemigatinib inhibited FGFR1-3 phosphorylation and signaling and decreased cell viability in cancer cell lines with activating FGFR amplifications and fusions that resulted in constitutive activation of FGFR signaling. Constitutive FGFR signaling can support the proliferation and survival of malignant cells. Pemigatinib exhibited anti-tumor activity in mouse xenograft models of human tumors with FGFR1, FGFR2, or FGFR3 alterations resulting in constitutive FGFR activation including a patient-derived xenograft model of cholangiocarcinoma that expressed an oncogenic FGFR2 Transformer-2 beta homolog (TRA2b) fusion protein.	PEMAZYRE is a kinase inhibitor indicated for the treatment of adults with previously treated, unresectable locally advanced or metastatic cholangiocarcinoma with a fibroblast growth factor receptor 2 (FGFR2) fusion or other rearrangement as detected by an FDA-approved test. This indication is approved under accelerated approval based on overall response rate and duration of response. Continued approval for this indication may be contingent upon verification and description of clinical benefit in a confirmatory trial(s).
Pexidartinib/ Turalio	Multiple kinases. Pexidartinib is a small molecule	The treatment of adult patients with symptomatic tenosynovial giant cell tumor (TGCT)

	tyrosine kinase inhibitor that targets colony stimulating factor 1 receptor (CSF1R), KIT proto-oncogene receptor tyrosine kinase (KIT), and FMS-like tyrosine kinase 3 (FLT3) harboring an internal tandem duplication (ITD) mutation. Overexpression of the CSF1R ligand promotes cell proliferation and accumulation in the synovium. In vitro, pexidartinib inhibited proliferation of cell lines dependent on CSF1R and ligand-induced autophosphorylation of CSF1R. Pexidartinib also inhibited the proliferation of a CSF1R dependent cell line in vivo.	associated with severe morbidity or functional limitations and not amenable to improvement with surgery.
Ponatinib/ Iclusig	ABL Ponatinib inhibited the in vitro tyrosine kinase activity of ABL and T315I mutant ABL with IC50 concentrations of 0.4 and 2.0 nM, respectively. Ponatinib inhibited the in vitro activity of additional kinases with IC50 concentrations between 0.1 and 20 nM, including members of the VEGFR, PDGFR, FGFR, EPH receptors and SRC families of kinases, and KIT, RET, TIE2, and FLT3. Ponatinib inhibited the in vitro viability of cells expressing native or mutant BCR-ABL, including T315I. In mice, treatment with ponatinib reduced the size of tumors expressing native or T315I mutant BCR-ABL when compared to controls.	Iclusig is a kinase inhibitor indicated for the: 1. Treatment of adult patients with chronic phase, accelerated phase, or blast phase chronic myeloid leukemia (CML) or Ph+ ALL for whom no other tyrosine kinase inhibitor (TKI) therapy is indicated. 2. Treatment of adult patients with T315I-positive CML (chronic phase, accelerated phase, or blast phase) or T315I-positive Philadelphia chromosome positive acute lymphoblastic leukemia (Ph+ ALL)
Pralsetinib/Gavreto	Kinase inhibitor of wild-type RET and oncogenic RET fusions and mutations.	For the treatment of adult patients with metastatic RET fusion-positive non-small cell lung cancer (NSCLC) as detected by an FDA approved test
Regorafenib/ Tafinlar	VEGFR1/2/3 Regorafenib is a small molecule inhibitor of multiple membrane-bound and intracellular kinases involved in normal cellular functions and in pathologic processes such as oncogenesis, tumor angiogenesis, and maintenance of the tumor microenvironment. In in vitro biochemical or cellular assays, regorafenib or its major human active metabolites M-2 and M-5 inhibited the activity of RET, VEGFR1, VEGFR2, VEGFR3, KIT, PDGFR-	Metastatic colorectal cancer (CRC) who have been previously treated with fluoropyrimidine-, oxaliplatin- and irinotecan-based chemotherapy, an anti-VEGF therapy, and, if KRAS wild type, an anti-EGFR therapy

	alpha, PDGFR-beta, FGFR1, FGFR2, TIE2, DDR2, Trk2A, Eph2A, RAF-1, BRAF, BRAFV600E , SAPK2, PTK5, and Abl at concentrations of regorafenib that have been achieved clinically. In in vivo models, regorafenib demonstrated anti-angiogenic activity in a rat tumor model, and inhibition of tumor growth as well as anti-metastatic activity in several mouse xenograft models including some for human colorectal carcinoma.	
Ribociclib/ Kisqali	CDK4/6 Ribociclib is an inhibitor of cyclin-dependent kinase (CDK) 4 and 6. These kinases are activated upon binding to Dcyclins and play a crucial role in signalling pathways which lead to cell cycle progression and cellular proliferation. The cyclin D-CDK4/6 complex regulates cell cycle progression through phosphorylation of the retinoblastoma protein (pRb). In vitro, ribociclib decreased pRb phosphorylation leading to arrest in the G1 phase of the cell cycle and reduced cell proliferation in non-Hodgkin's lymphoma cell lines. In vivo, treatment with single agent ribociclib in a rat xenograft model with human tumor cells led to decreased tumor volumes, which correlated with inhibition of pRb phosphorylation.	IBRANCE is a kinase inhibitor indicated for the treatment of adult patients with hormone receptor (HR)-positive, human epidermal growth factor receptor 2 (HER2)-negative advanced or metastatic breast cancer in combination with: • an aromatase inhibitor as initial endocrine-based therapy in postmenopausal women or in men; or • fulvestrant in patients with disease progression following endocrine therapy
Ripretinib/ QINLOCK™	KIT, PDGFRA	QINLOCK is a kinase inhibitor indicated for the treatment of adult patients with advanced gastrointestinal stromal tumor (GIST) who have received prior treatment with 3 or more kinase inhibitors, including imatinib. Ripretinib is a tyrosine kinase inhibitor that inhibits KIT proto-oncogene receptor tyrosine kinase (KIT) and platelet derived growth factor receptor A (PDGFRA) kinase, including wild type, primary, and secondary mutations. Ripretinib also inhibits other kinases in vitro, such as PDGFRB, TIE2, VEGFR2, and BRAF.
Ruxolitinib/ Jakafi	JAK1/2/3,Tyk Ruxolitinib, a kinase inhibitor, inhibits	Jakafi is a kinase inhibitor indicated for treatment of patients with intermediate or high-risk

	Janus Associated Kinases (JAKs) JAK1 and JAK2 which mediate the signalling of a number of cytokines and growth factors that are important for hematopoiesis and immune function. JAK signalling involves recruitment of STATs (signal transducers and activators of transcription) to cytokine receptors, activation and subsequent localization of STATs to the nucleus leading to modulation of gene expression. Myelofibrosis (MF) is a myeloproliferative neoplasm (MPN) known to be associated with dysregulated JAK1 and JAK2 signalling. In a mouse model of JAK2V617F-positive MPN, oral administration of ruxolitinib prevented splenomegaly, preferentially decreased JAK2V617F mutant cells in the spleen and decreased circulating inflammatory cytokines (eg, TNF-α, IL-6).	myelofibrosis, including primary myelofibrosis, post-polycythemia vera myelofibrosis and post-essential thrombocythemia myelofibrosis
Selpercatinib/ RETEVMO	RET Selpercatinib is a kinase inhibitor. Selpercatinib inhibited wild-type RET and multiple mutated RET isoforms as well as VEGFR1 and VEGFR3 with IC50 values ranging from 0.92 nM to 67.8 nM. In other enzyme assays, selpercatinib also inhibited FGFR 1, 2, and 3 at higher concentrations that were still clinically achievable. In cellular assays, selpercatinib inhibited RET at approximately 60-fold lower concentrations than FGFR1 and 2 and approximately 8-fold lower concentration than VEGFR3. Certain point mutations in RET or chromosomal rearrangements involving in-frame fusions of RET with various partners can result in constitutively activated chimeric RET fusion proteins that can act as oncogenic drivers by promoting cell proliferation of tumor cell lines. In in vitro and in vivo tumor models, selpercatinib demonstrated anti-tumor activity in cells harboring constitutive activation of RET protein resulting from gene fusions and mutations, including CCDC6-RET, KIF5B-RET, RET V804M, and RET M918T. In addition, selpercatinib showed anti-tumor activity in mice intracranially implanted with a patient-derived RET fusion positive	RETEVMO is a kinase inhibitor indicated for the treatment of: • Adult patients with metastatic RET fusion-positive non-small cell lung cancer (NSCLC)1 • Adult and pediatric patients 12 years of age and older with advanced or metastatic RET-mutant medullary thyroid cancer (MTC) who require systemic therapy • Adult and pediatric patients 12 years of age and older with advanced or metastatic RET fusion-positive thyroid cancer who require systemic therapy and who are radioactive iodine-refractory (if radioactive iodine is appropriate). 1 This indication is approved under accelerated approval based on overall response rate and duration of response. Continued approval for this indication may be contingent upon verification and description of clinical benefit in confirmatory Selpercatinib is a kinase inhibitor. Selpercatinib inhibited wild-type RET and multiple mutated RET isoforms as well as VEGFR1 and VEGFR3 with IC50 values ranging from 0.92 nM to 67.8 nM. In other enzyme assays, selpercatinib also

	tumor.	inhibited FGFR 1, 2, and 3 at higher concentrations that were still clinically achievable. In cellular assays, selpercatinib inhibited RET at approximately 60-fold lower concentrations than FGFR1 and 2 and approximately 8-fold lower concentration than VEGFR3. Certain point mutations in RET or chromosomal rearrangements involving in-frame fusions of RET with various partners can result in constitutively activated chimeric RET fusion proteins that can act as oncogenic drivers by promoting cell proliferation of tumor cell lines. In in vitro and in vivo tumor models, selpercatinib demonstrated anti-tumor activity in cells harboring constitutive activation of RET protein resulting from gene fusions and mutations, including CCDC6-RET, KIF5B-RET, RET V804M, and RET M918T. In addition, selpercatinib showed Reference ID: 4605720 anti-tumor activity in mice intracranially implanted with a patient-derived RET fusion positive tumor trial(s).
Selumetinib/ KOSELUGO	MEK1/2 Selumetinib is an inhibitor of mitogen-activated protein kinase kinases 1 and 2 (MEK1/2). MEK1/2 proteins are upstream regulators of the extracellular signal-related kinase (ERK) pathway. Both MEK and ERK are critical components of the RAS-regulated RAF-MEK-ERK pathway, which is often activated in different types of cancers. In genetically modified mouse models of NF1 that generate neurofibromas that recapitulate the genotype and phenotype of human NF1, oral dosing of selumetinib inhibited ERK phosphorylation, and reduced neurofibroma numbers, volume, and proliferation.	KOSELUGO is a kinase inhibitor indicated for the treatment of pediatric patients 2 years of age and older with neurofibromatosis type 1 (NF1) who have symptomatic, inoperable plexiform neurofibromas (PN).
Sorafenib/ Nexavar	VEGFR1/2/3 Sorafenib has been shown to inhibit multiple intracellular (c-CRAF, BRAF and mutant BRAF) and cell surface kinases (KIT, FLT- 3, RET, RET/PTC, VEGFR-1, VEGFR- 2, VEGFR- 3, and PDGFR-ß). Several	Treatment of 1.Unresectable hepatocellular carcinoma (HCC) 2. Advanced renal cell carcinoma (RCC) 3. Locally recurrent or metastatic,

	of these kinases are thought to be involved in tumor cell signalling, angiogenesis and apoptosis. Sorafenib inhibited tumor growth of HCC, RCC, and DTC human tumor xenografts in immunocompromised mice. Reductions in tumor angiogenesis were seen in models of HCC and RCC upon sorafenib treatment, and increases in tumor apoptosis were observed in models of HCC, RCC, and DTC.	progressive, differentiated thyroid carcinoma (DTC) refractory to radioactive iodine treatment
Sunitinib/ Sutent	Multiple kinases. Sunitinib is a small molecule that inhibits multiple receptor tyrosine kinases (RTKs), some of which are implicated in tumor growth, pathologic angiogenesis, and metastatic progression of cancer. Sunitinib was evaluated for its inhibitory activity against a variety of kinases (>80 kinases) and was identified as an inhibitor of platelet-derived growth factor receptors (PDGFRα and PDGFRβ), vascular endothelial growth factor receptors (VEGFR1, VEGFR2 and VEGFR3), stem cell factor receptor (KIT), Fms-like tyrosine kinase-3 (FLT3), colony stimulating factor receptor Type 1 (CSF-1R), and the glial cell-line derived neurotrophic factor receptor (RET). Sunitinib inhibited the phosphorylation of multiple RTKs (PDGFRβ, VEGFR2, KIT) in tumor xenografts expressing RTK targets in vivo and demonstrated inhibition of tumor growth or tumor regression and/or inhibited metastases in some experimental models of cancer. Sunitinib demonstrated the ability to inhibit growth of tumor cells expressing dysregulated target RTKs (PDGFR, RET, or KIT) in vitro and to inhibit PDGFRβ- and VEGFR2-dependent tumor angiogenesis in vivo.	The treatment of: 1. Gastrointestinal stromal tumor (GIST) after disease progression on or intolerance to imatinib mesylate. 2. Advanced renal cell carcinoma (RCC). 3. Progressive, well-differentiated pancreatic neuroendocrine tumors (pNET) in patients with unresectable locally advanced or metastatic disease
Tofacitinib/ Xeljanz/ Xeljanz XR	JAK Tofacitinib is a Janus kinase (JAK) inhibitor. JAKs are intracellular enzymes which transmit signals arising from cytokine or growth factor-receptor interactions on the cellular membrane to influence cellular processes of hematopoiesis and immune cell function. Within the signalling pathway, JAKs	1. Rheumatoid arthritis: XELJANZ/XELJANZ XR is indicated for the treatment of adult patients with moderately to severely active rheumatoid arthritis who have had an inadequate response or intolerance to methotrexate. It may be used as monotherapy or in combination with methotrexate or other non-biologic disease-

	phosphorylate and activate Signal Transducers and Activators of Transcription (STATs) which modulate intracellular activity including gene expression. Tofacitinib modulates the signalling pathway at the point of JAKs, preventing the phosphorylation and activation of 26 Reference ID: 4467787 STATs. JAK enzymes transmit cytokine signalling through pairing of JAKs (e.g., JAK1/JAK3, JAK1/JAK2, JAK1/TyK2, JAK2 /JAK2). Tofacitinib inhibited the in vitro activities of JAK1/JAK2, JAK1/JAK3, and JAK2/JAK2 combinations with IC50 of 406, 56, and 1377 nM, respectively. However, the relevance of specific JAK combinations to therapeutic effectiveness is not known.	modifying antrheumatic drugs (DMARDs). ○ Limitations of use: use of XELJANZ/XELJANZ XR in combination with biologic DMARDs or potent immunosuppressants such as azathioprine and cyclosporine is not recommended. 2. Psoriatic arthritis: XELJANZ/XELJANZ XR is indicated for the treatment of adult patients with active psoriatic arthritis who have had an inadequate response or intolerance to methotrexate or other disease-modifying anti-rheumatic drugs (DMARDs). ○ Limitations of use: use of XELJANZ/XELJANZ XR in combination with biologic DMARDs or potent immunosuppressants such as azathioprine and cyclosporine is not recommended. 3. Ulcerative colitis: XELJANZ is indicated for the treatment of adult patients with moderately to severely active ulcerative colitis (UC), who have had an inadequate response or who are intolerant to TNF blockers. ○ Limitations of use: use of XELJANZ in combination with biological therapies for UC or with potent immunosuppressants such as azathioprine and cyclosporine is not recommended.
Trametinib/ Mekinist	MEK1/2 Trametinib is a reversible inhibitor of mitogen-activated extracellular signal-regulated kinase 1 (MEK1) and MEK2 activation and of MEK1 and MEK2 kinase activity. MEK proteins are upstream regulators of the extracellular signal-related kinase (ERK) pathway, which promotes cellular proliferation. BRAF V600E mutations result in constitutive activation of the BRAF pathway which includes MEK1 and MEK2. Trametinib inhibits cell growth of various BRAF V600 mutation-positive tumors in vitro and in vivo. Trametinib and dabrafenib target two different	MEKINIST is a kinase inhibitor indicated as a single agent for the treatment of patients with unresectable or metastatic melanoma with BRAF V600E or V600K mutations as detected by an FDA-approved test. MEKINIST is indicated, in combination with dabrafenib, for: • the treatment of patients with unresectable or metastatic melanoma with BRAF V600E or V600K mutations as detected by an FDA-approved test. • the adjuvant treatment of patients with melanoma with

	kinases in the RAS/RAF/MEK/ERK pathway. Use of trametinib and dabrafenib in combination resulted in greater growth inhibition of BRAF V600 mutation-positive tumor cell lines in vitro and prolonged inhibition of tumor growth in BRAF V600 mutation positive tumor xenografts compared with either drug alone.	BRAF V600E or V600K mutations, as detected by an FDA-approved test, and involvement of lymph node(s), following complete resection. • the treatment of patients with metastatic non-small cell lung cancer (NSCLC) with BRAF V600E mutation as detected by an FDA-approved test. Limitation of Use: MEKINIST is not indicated for treatment of patients with melanoma who have progressed on prior BRAF-inhibitor therapy
Tucatinib/TUKYSA	HER2 Tucatinib is a tyrosine kinase inhibitor of HER2. In vitro, tucatinib inhibits phosphorylation of HER2 and HER3, resulting in inhibition of downstream MAPK and AKT signaling and cell proliferation, and showed antitumor activity in HER2 expressing tumor cells. In vivo, tucatinib inhibited the growth of HER2 expressing tumors. The combination of tucatinib and trastuzumab showed increased anti-tumor activity in vitro and in vivo compared to either drug alone.	TUKYSA is a kinase inhibitor indicated in combination with trastuzumab and capecitabine for treatment of adult patients with advanced unresectable or metastatic HER2-positive breast cancer, including patients with brain metastases, who have received one or more prior anti-HER2-based regimens in the metastatic setting
Vemurafenib/ Zelboraf	B-Raf Vemurafenib is a low molecular weight, orally available inhibitor of some mutated forms of BRAF serine-threonine kinase, including BRAF V600E. Vemurafenib also inhibits other kinases in vitro such as CRAF, ARAF, wild-type BRAF, SRMS, ACK1, MAP4K5, and FGR at similar concentrations. Some mutations in the BRAF gene including V600E result in constitutively activated BRAF proteins, which can cause cell proliferation in the absence of growth factors that would normally be required for proliferation. Vemurafenib has anti-tumor effects in cellular and animal models of melanoma with mutated BRAF V600E.	ZELBORAF® is a kinase inhibitor indicated for the treatment of patients with unresectable or metastatic melanoma with BRAF V600E mutation as detected by an FDA-approved test. Limitation of Use: ZELBORAF is not indicated for treatment of patients with wild-type BRAF melanoma.
Upadacitinib/Rinvaq	Janus kinase inhibitor	The treatment of adults with moderately to severely active rheumatoid arthritis who have had an inadequate response or intolerance to methotrexate.

		Limitation of use: use of RINVOQ in combination with other JAK inhibitors, biologic DMARDs, or with potent immunosuppressants such as azathioprine and cyclosporine is not recommended

[1]Ogden Carr Bruton (1908 - 2003) was an American pediatrician

Summary of treatments derived from of the biological discoveries in the last 70 years

94 monoclonal antibodies (including biosimilars) and 59 small molecule protein kinase inhibitors are now FDA-approved for therapeutic purposes. Additional classes of therapeutics include new cellular therapies including gene-modified cellular therapies and gene therapies that have also been FDA-approved for therapeutic use All these agents will be described in detail in each book on diseases for which they have been approved.

This book deals with their use in **non-melanoma skin cancers.** It is one in a series of books on the impact of targeted biological and specifically designed therapeutic agents across the whole field of medicine in a series called Medicine 2020.

4. The biology of non-malignant human cells

To fully understand how these new therapeutic agents work it is useful to understand how cells work – in particular what signalling pathways they use. Normal cells and cells in tissues affected by non- diseases use signalling pathways often different from those used by cells.

All human cells are derived from a single totipotent stem cell which is produced by the fusion of a single sperm with a single ovum. This totipotent stem cell has all the genes on its chromosomes responsible for the future growth and development of the fetus, including reproductive capacity. Cell biology is concerned with the physiological properties, metabolic processes, signalling pathways, life cycle, chemical composition and interactions of cells with their environment. Cell biology involves genetics, biochemistry, molecular biology, immunology and cytochemistry. Human cells are eukaryotes - they contain organelles. The generalized structure of a eukaryotic cell is shown in Figure 2.

Figure 2. A diagram of a mammalian cell

This image has been released into the public domain by its author, LadyofHats (Mariana Ruiz). Source: own work using Adobe Illustrator. Image renamed from Image:Animal cell structure.svg. https://commons.wikimedia.org/wiki/File:Animal_cell_structure_en.svg. No changes have been made to this image.

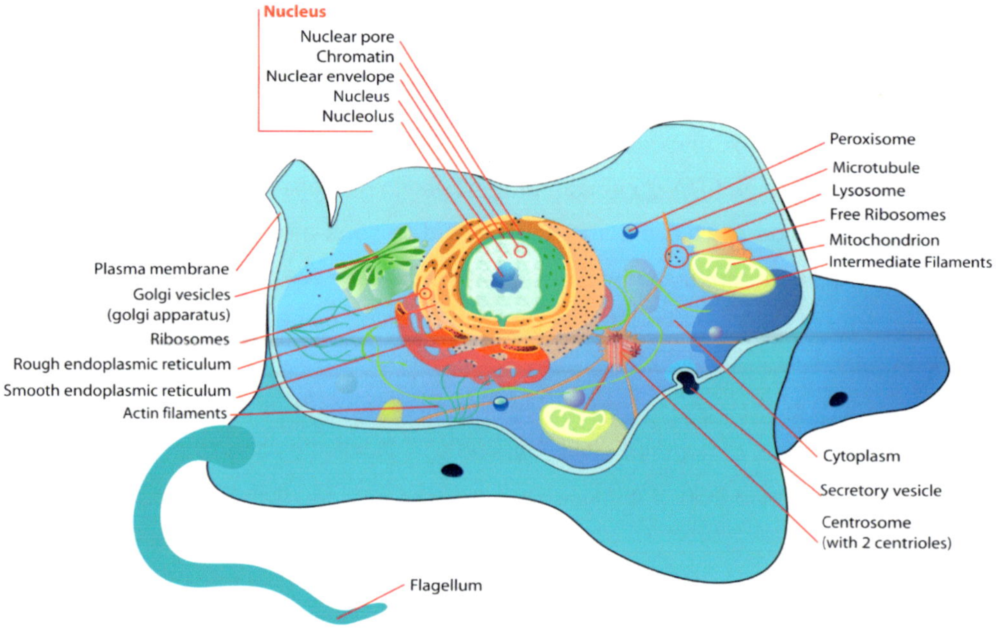

Most of the processes of eukaryotic cells are performed by a mixture of small organic molecules, inorganic ions, hormones and water. Approximately 75-85% of the cell's volume is due to water making it an indispensable solvent as a result of its polarity and structure. The shape of cells are generally round and spherical or oval.

The main constituents of the cell include proteins and lipids which are either free-flowing or membrane-bound, along with different internal compartments known as organelles. The cytoplasm is all of the material within a cell, enclosed by the cell membrane, except for the cell nucleus. The material inside the nucleus and contained within the nuclear membrane is termed the nucleoplasm. A cell's DNA, contained on the cell's chromosomes, is located within the cell's nucleus. The main components of the cytoplasm are cytosol – a gel-like substance, the organelles – the cell's internal sub-structures - and various cytoplasmic inclusions. Cell are composed of hydrophilic and hydrophobic regions. The hydrophilic regions of the cell are on both the inside and outside of the cell, while the hydrophobic regions are within the phospholipid bilayer of the cell membrane. A diagram of a mammalian cell membrane is shown in Figure 3. This shows the detailed diagram of lipid bilayer cell membrane. The cell membrane, also called the plasma membrane or plasmalemma, biological molecules, primarily proteins and lipids, which are involved in a vast array of cellular processes. It also serves as the attachment point for both the intracellular cytoskeleton and, if present, the cell wall.

Figure 3.

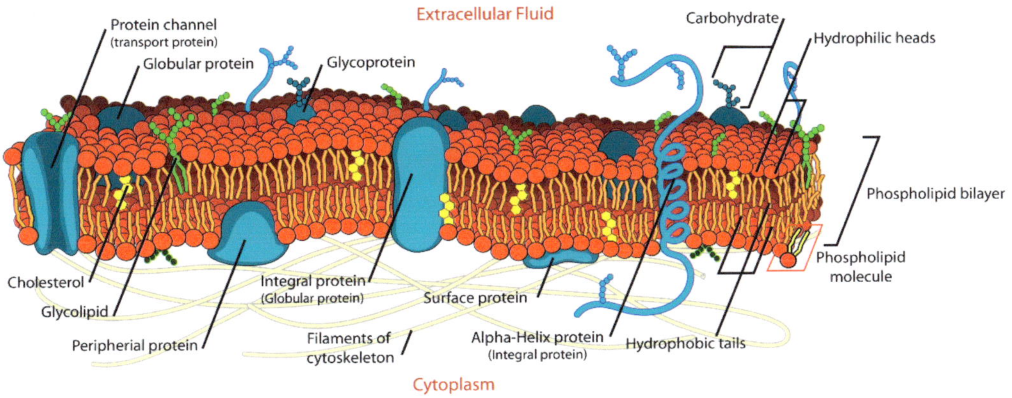

This image, reproduced here from Wikimedia Commons, has been released into the public domain by its author, LadyofHats (Mariana Ruiz). Source: Own work. Image renamed from File:Cell membrane detailed diagram.svg.
https://commons.wikimedia.org/wiki/File:Cell_membrane_detailed_diagram_en.svg. No changes have been made to this image.

In order for molecules to participate in reactions within the cell, they need to be able to cross this membrane layer to get into the cell. They accomplish this process of gaining access to the cell via osmotic pressure, diffusion, concentration gradients, and membrane channels. Inside the cell are extensive internal suB cellular membrane-bounded compartments called organelles.

Figure 4. Some of the cell surface proteins and internal signalling pathways of a normal human cell.

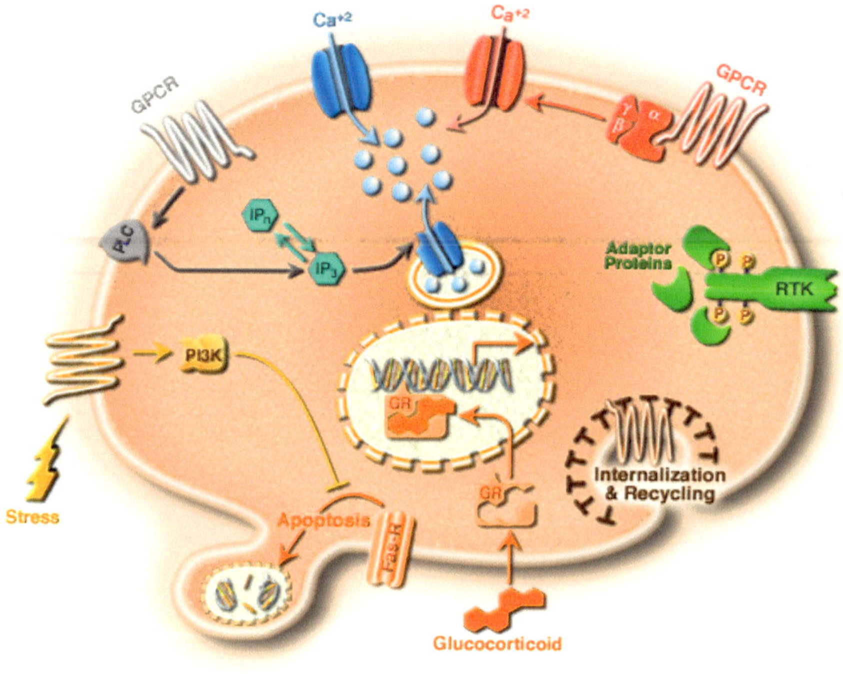

Cell growth pertains to the increase in the number of cells present in an organism as it grows and develops; in order for the organism to grow the number of cells present must increase. To enable cell growth and development the cell goes through the steps of the cell cycle: DNA replication, cell division, regeneration, specialization, and cell death. The cell cycle is divided into four distinct phases, G1, S, G2, and M. The G phases (cell growth) make up approximately 95% of the cycle. After proliferation cells then differentiate to become specialized in order to form specialized tissues, then organs and ultimately systems. The G phases along with the S phase – DNA replication, damage and repair - are considered to be the interphase portion of the cycle. While the M phase (mitosis and cytokinesis) is the cell division portion of the cycle. The cell cycle is regulated by a series of signalling factors and complexes such as cyclin-dependent kinases and p53. When the cell has completed its growth process, and if it is found to be damaged or altered, it undergoes cell death, either by apoptosis or necrosis, in order to eliminate the threat it can cause to the organism's survival. Some of the main cell surface proteins and internal signalling processes are shown in Figure 3.

Essential cell processes include

- Active transport and passive transport – the movement of molecules into and out of cells
- Adhesion - holding cells and tissues together
- Cell movement - chemotaxis, contraction and cilia
- Cell signalling - regulation of cell behaviour by signals from outside and inside the cell
- Division – the process by which cells reproduce either by mitosis (to produce clones of the parent cell) or meiosis (to produce haploid gametes either male [sperm)] or female [ova]) dependent on the gender of the organism
- DNA repair - cell death and cell senescence
- Metabolism - glycolysis, respiration, photosynthesis, and chemosynthesis
- Signal transduction - the process by which the activities in the cell are regulated
- Transcription and mRNA splicing - gene expression

Three of the most important processes – signal transduction, gene expression and apoptosis (also known as programmed cell death) - are described furtherl below. Some of the most important pathways for understanding the basis of targeted therapies, such as the pathways for angiogenesis, interkeukin (IL) 4, IL-12 and IL-23 and the TNF pathways are described in chapters dealing with the therapeutic use of molecules involved in these pathways.

Signal transduction and cell signalling pathways

Signal transduction is the process by which a chemical or physical signal is transmitted through a cell as a series of molecular events, most commonly protein phosphorylation catalyzed by protein kinases, which ultimately results in a cellular response. Proteins responsible for detecting stimuli such as ligands are termed receptors The changes elicited by ligand binding to a receptor give rise to a biochemical cascade otherwise known as a signalling path. A simplified representation of major signal transduction pathways in mammals is shown in Figure 5.

Figure 5

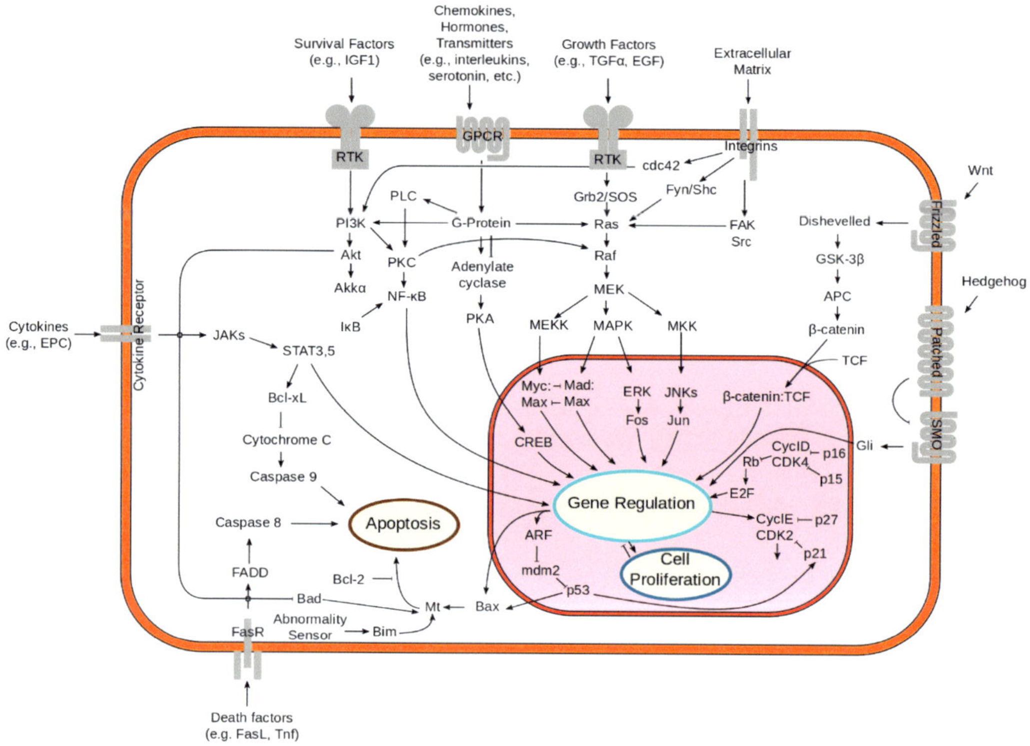

Figure 5. A simplified representation of major signal transduction pathways in mammals. This image is reproduced here from Wikimedia Commons since permission has been granted by its creator, Cybertory, to copy, distribute and/or modify this document under the terms of the GNU Free Documentation License, Version 1.2 or any later version published by the Free Software Foundation. Author: By Cybertory - This file was derived from: Signal transduction v1.png, CC BY-SA 3.0, https://commons.wikimedia.org/w/index.php?curid=12081090; https://en.wikipedia.org/wiki/Creative_Commons_license. No changes have been made to the image

When signalling pathways interact with one another they form networks, which allow cellular responses to be coordinated, often by combinatorial signalling events. At the molecular level, such responses include changes in the transcription or translation of genes, and post-translational and conformational changes in proteins, as well as changes in their location. These molecular events are the basic mechanisms controlling cell growth, proliferation, metabolism and many other processes. In multicellular organisms, signal transduction pathways have evolved to regulate cell communication in a wide variety of ways.

Each component (or node) of a signalling pathway is classified according to the role it plays with respect to the initial stimulus. Ligands are termed first messengers, while receptors are the signal transducers, which then activate primary effectors. Such effectors are often linked to second messengers, which can activate secondary effectors, and so on. Depending on the efficiency of the nodes, a signal can be amplified (a concept known as signal gain), so that one signalling molecule can generate a response involving hundreds to millions of molecules With the advent of computational biology, the analysis of signalling pathways and networks has become an essential tool to understand cellular functions and disease, including signalling rewiring mechanisms underlying responses to acquired drug resistance.

Ligands

The majority of signal transduction pathways involve the binding of signalling molecules, known as ligands, to receptors that trigger events inside the cell. The binding of a signalling molecule with a receptor causes a change in the conformation of the receptor, known as receptor activation. Most ligands are soluble molecules from the extracellular medium which bind to cell surface receptors. These include growth factors, cytokines and neurotransmitters. Components of the extracellular matrix such as fibronectin and hyaluronan can also bind to such receptors (integrins and CD44, respectively). In addition, some molecules such as steroid hormones are lipid-soluble and thus cross the plasma membrane to reach nuclear receptors.

Some receptors such as HER2/neu are capable of ligand-independent activation when overexpressed or mutated. This leads to constitutive activation of the pathway, which may or may not be overturned by compensation mechanisms. In the case of HER2, which acts as a dimerization partner of other EGFRs, constitutive activation leads to hyperproliferation and cancer – primarily some cases of breast cancer and gastric cancer (HER2/neu is also known as receptor tyrosine-protein kinase erbB-2, CD340, proto-oncogene Neu and ERBB2). A ribbon diagram of the Fab fragment of trastuzumab, a monoclonal antibody, bound to the extracellulardomain of HER2 is shown in Figure 6.

Figure 6.

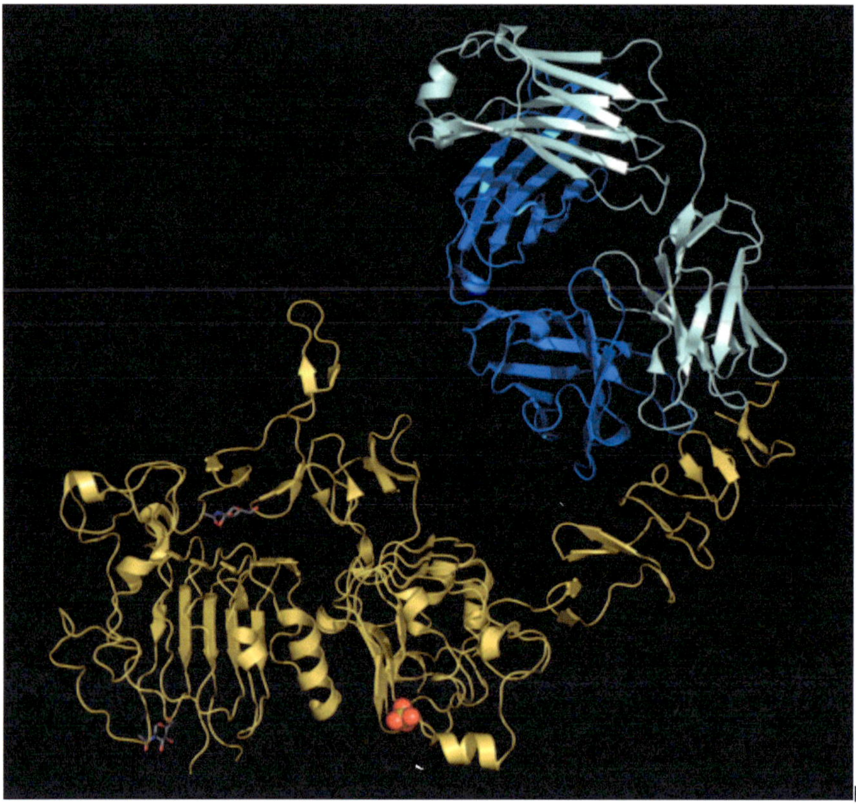

Figure 6

Figure 6. Ribbon diagram of the Fab fragment of trastuzumab, a monoclonal antibody, bound to the extracellular domain of HER2. Legend: ▮ Trastuzumab Fab fragment, heavy chain ▯ ; Trastuzumab Fab fragment, light chain ▯ ; HER2, extracellular domain This image, reproduced here from Wikimedia Commons, is in the public domain because its creator, Fvasconcellos, has placed it there. https://commons.wikimedia.org/wiki/File:Trastuzumab_Fab-HER2_complex_1N8Z.png#/media/File:Trastuzumab_Fab-HER2_complex_1N8Z.png; https://commons.wikimedia.org/wiki/User:Fvasconcellos. Created using Accelrys DS Visualizer Pro 1.6 and GIMP. More information: Cho HS, Mason K, Ramyar KX, et al. (2003). "Structure of the extracellular region of HER2 alone and in complex with the Herceptin Fab". Nature 421 (6924): 756–60. PMID 12610629. doi:10.1038/nature01392. No changes have been made to this image.

Extracellular receptors, ligand binding, messengers and adaptor proteins

Extracellular receptors are integral transmembrane proteins that span the plasma membrane (Figure 2) of the cell, with one part of the receptor on the outside of the cell and the other on the inside. Signal transduction occurs as a result of a ligand binding to the outside region of the receptor (the ligand does not pass through the membrane). Ligand-receptor binding induces a change in the conformation of the inside part of the receptor, a process sometimes called "receptor activation". This results in either the activation of an enzyme domain of the receptor or the exposure of a binding site for other intracellular signalling proteins within the cell, eventually propagating the signal through the cytoplasm (Figure 5).

In mammalian cells most intracellular proteins activated by a ligand/receptor interaction possess an enzymatic activity; examples include tyrosine kinases and phosphatases. Often such enzymes are covalently linked to the receptor. Some of them create second messengers such as cyclic AMP and IP3, the latter controlling the release of intracellular calcium stores into the cytoplasm. Other activated proteins interact with adaptor proteins (an example is shown Figure 4) that facilitate signalling protein interactions and coordination of signalling complexes necessary to respond to a particular stimulus. Enzymes and adaptor proteins are both responsive to various second messenger molecules.

Many adaptor proteins and enzymes activated as part of signal transduction possess specialized protein domains that bind to specific secondary messenger molecules. For example, calcium ions bind to the EF hand domains of calmodulin, allowing it to bind and activate calmodulin-dependent kinase.

The following major extracellular receptor/ligand binding pathways will be discussed in more detail below:

- G protein-coupled receptors
- Tyrosine, seronine/threonine- and histidine-specific protein kinases
- Integrins
- Toll-like receptors

- Ligand-gated ion binding channels

G proteins, also known as guanine nucleotide-binding proteins, are a family of proteins that act as molecular switches inside cells, and are involved in transmitting signals from a variety of stimuli outside a cell to its interior. Their activity is regulated by factors that control their ability to bind to and hydrolyze guanosine triphosphate (GTP) to guanosine diphosphate (GDP). When they are bound to GTP, they are 'on', and, when they are bound to GDP, they are 'off'.

They possess seven transmembrane domains and are linked to a heterotrimeric G protein. A ribbon diagram of a G protein is shown in Figure 7. Beta and gamma subunits of G-protein are shown by blue and red, respectively, in the phosducin-transducin beta-gamma complex. (Phosducin binds tightly to the beta gamma subunits (Gt beta gamma) of the heterotrimeric G protein transducin, preventing Gt beta gamma reassociation with Gt alpha-GDP and thereby inhibiting the G-protein cycle).

Figure 7. Ribbon diagram of a G protein

This image, reproduced here from Wikimedia Commons, has been released into the public domain by its creator, Andrei Lomize, has placed it there. By Andrei Lomize - Own work, Public Domain,

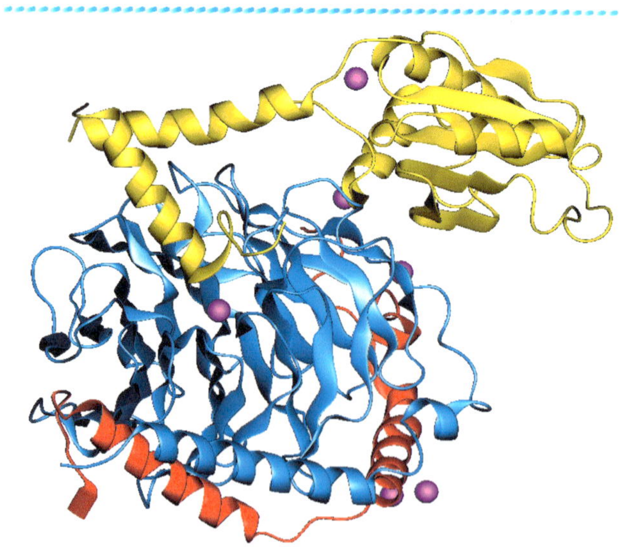

Tyrosine and seronine/threonine-specific protein kinases

Receptor tyrosine kinases (RTKs) are transmembrane proteins with an intracellular kinase domain and an extracellular domain that binds ligands (Figure 4); examples include growth factor receptors such as the insulin receptor. To perform signal transduction, RTKs need to form dimers in the plasma membrane. The dimer is stabilized by ligands binding to the receptor. The interaction between the cytoplasmic domains stimulates the autophosphorylation of tyrosine residues within the intracellular kinase domains of the RTKs, causing conformational changes. Subsequent to this, the receptors' kinase domains are activated, initiating phosphorylation signalling cascades of downstream cytoplasmic molecules that facilitate various cellular processes such as cell differentiation and metabolism. Many serine/threonine and dual-specificity protein kinases are important for signal transduction, either acting downstream of receptor tyrosine kinases, or as membrane-embedded or cell-soluble versions in their own right. The process of signal transduction involves around 560 known protein kinases and pseudokinanases, encoded by the human kinome. The kinome of an organism is the complete set of protein kinases encoded in its genome.

As is the case with GPCRs, proteins that bind GTP play a major role in signal transduction from the activated RTK into the cell. In this case, the G proteins are members of the Ras, Rho (see Figure 4 above), and Raf families, referred to collectively as small G proteins. They act as molecular switches usually tethered to membranes by isoprenyl groups linked to their carboxyl ends. Upon activation, they assign proteins to specific membrane subdomains where they participate in signalling. Activated RTKs in turn activate small G proteins that activate guanine nucleotide exchange factors such as SOS1. Once activated, these exchange factors can activate more small G proteins, thus amplifying the receptor's initial signal. The mutation of certain RTK genes, as with that of GPCRs, can result in the expression of receptors that exist in a constitutively activated state. Such mutated genes may act as oncogenes. An example is the BCR-ABL gene, which is translated to the BCR-ABL protein, a growth factor responsible for the development of chronic myeloid leukemia (CML). The first tyrosine kinase inhibitor developed that was therapeutically successful is imatinib, now routinely used as first-line treatment of CML, obviating the need in many cases of the only curative treatment for CML –

allogeneic hematopoietic stem cell transplantaion, a procedure that had a treatment-related mortality of 20-30%.

Integrins

Integrins are produced by a wide variety of cells. They play a role in cell attachment to other cells and the extracellular matrix and in the transduction of signals from extracellular matrix components such as fibronectin and collagen (Figure 8).

Figure 8. An overview of integrin-mediated signal transduction, adapted from Hehlgens et al. (2007).

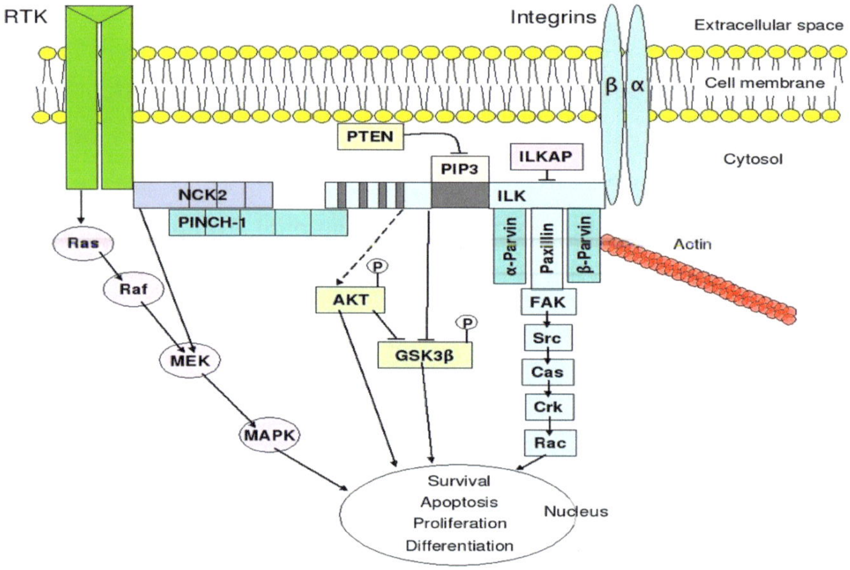

This image, reproduced here from Wikimedia Commons, has been released into the public domain by its author, K.murphy at English Wikipedia. https://commons.wikimedia.org/wiki/File:Integrin_sig_trans_overview.jpeg. Original source: Hehlgans S, Haase M, Cordes N (Jan 2007). "Signalling via integrins: implications for cell survival and anticancer strategies". Biochimica et Biophysica Acta. 1775 (1): 163–80. doi:10.1016/j.bbcan.2006.09.001. PMID 17084981.

Ligand binding to the extracellular domain of integrins changes the protein's conformation, clustering it at the cell membrane to initiate signal transduction. Integrins lack kinase activity; hence, integrin-mediated signal transduction is achieved through a variety of intracellular protein kinases and adaptor molecules, the main coordinator being integrin-linked kinase. As shown in Figure 7, cooperative integrin-RTK signalling determines the timing of cellular survival, apoptosis, proliferation and differentiation.

Toll-like receptors

When activated, toll-like receptors (TLRs) take adapter molecules within the cytoplasm of cells in order to propagate a signal.

Figure 9. Cellular signalling pathways activated by Toll-like receptors. Dashed grey lines represent unknown associations.

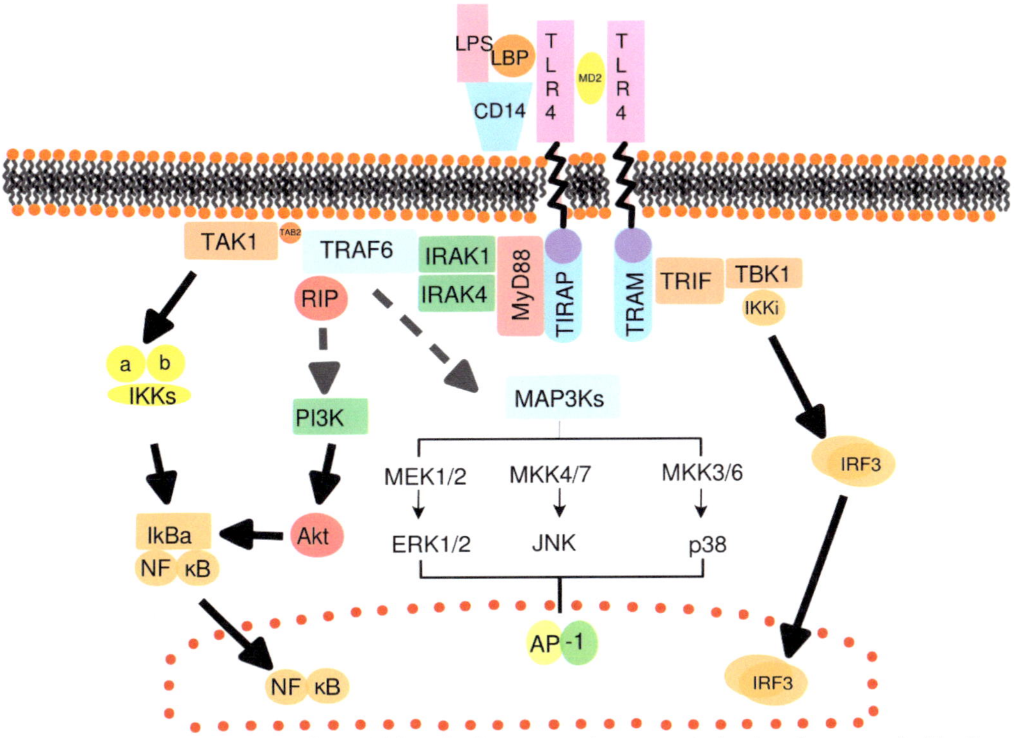

Four adaptor molecules are known to be involved in signalling. These are Myd88, TIRAP, TRIF, and TRAM. These adapter molecules activate other intracellular molecules such as IRAK1, IRAK4, TBK1, and IKKi that amplify the signal, eventually leading to the induction or suppression of genes that cause certain responses. Thousands of genes are activated by TLR signalling, implying that this method constitutes an important gateway for gene modulation.

Messenger systems

First messengers are the signalling molecules (hormones, neurotransmitters and paracrine/autocrine agents) that reach the cell from the extracellular fluid and bind to their specific receptors.

Second messengers are the substances that enter the cytoplasm and act within the cell to trigger a response. Second messengers serve as chemical relays from the plasma membrane to the cytoplasm, thus carrying out intracellular signal transduction.

Calcium

The release of calcium ions from the endoplasmic reticulum (Figure 1) into the cytosol results in its binding to signalling proteins that are then activated. It is then sequestered in the smooth endoplasmic reticulum and the mitochondria (Figure 1). Calcium is used in many processes including muscle contraction, neurotransmitter release from nerve endings, and cell migration. The three main pathways that lead to its activation are GPCR pathways, RTK pathways, and gated ion channels. It regulates proteins either directly or by binding to an enzyme.

Cellular responses

Gene activations and metabolism alterations are examples of cellular responses to extracellular stimulation that require signal transduction. Gene activation leads to further cellular effects, since the products of responding genes include instigators of activation. Transcription factors produced as a result of a signal transduction cascade can activate even more genes. Hence, an initial stimulus can trigger the expression of a large number of genes, leading to physiological events. Examples are the increased uptake of glucose from the blood stream and the migration of neutrophils to sites of infection.

Mammalian cells require stimulation for cell division and survival. In the absence of growth factor, apoptosis (programmed cell death – see below) ensues. Such requirements for extracellular stimulation are necessary for controlling cell behavior.

Signal transduction pathways are perceived to be so central to biological processes that a large number of diseases are attributed to their dysregulation. Three basic types of signals determine cellular growth:

1. **Stimulatory signals (growth factors)**

Transcription-dependent response
Steroids are an example of this. They bind DNA, which needs to be transcribed. The produced mRNA needs to be translated, and the produced protein/peptide can undergo posttranslational modification (PMT).

Transcription-independent response
Epidermal growth factor (EGF) is an example. It binds to the epidermal growth factor receptor (EGFR), which causes dimerization and autophosphorylation of the EGFR, which in turn activates the intracellular signalling pathway.

2. **Inhibitory signals (cell-cell contact)**

3. **Permissive signals (cell-matrix interactions)**

The combination of these signals are integrated in an altered cytoplasmic machinery which leads to altered cell behaviour.

Major cell signalling pathways
The following are some of the major cell signalling pathways, demonstrating how ligands binding to their receptors can affect second messengers and eventually result in altered cellular responses.

- MAPK/ERK pathway: a pathway that couples intracellular responses to the binding of growth factors to cell surface receptors. This pathway is very complex and includes many protein components. In many cell types, activation of this pathway promotes cell division, and many forms of cancer are associated with aberrations in it.

- cAMP-dependent pathway: cAMP works by activating protein kinase A (PKA, cAMP-dependent protein kinase (Figure 11). Further effects depend mainly on cAMP-dependent protein kinase, which vary based on the type of cell involved.

- IP3/DAG pathway: PLC cleaves the phospholipid phosphatidylinositol 4,5-bisphosphate (PIP2), yielding diacyl glycerol (DAG) and inositol 1,4,5-triphosphate (IP3). DAG remains bound to the membrane, and IP3 is released as a soluble structure into the cytosol. IP3 then diffuses through the cytosol to bind to IP3 receptors, particular calcium channels in the endoplasmic reticulum (ER). These channels are specific to calcium and allow the passage of only calcium to move through. This causes the cytosolic concentration of calcium to increase, in turn precipitating a cascade of intracellular changes and activity. In addition, calcium and DAG together work to activate PKC, which then phosphorylates other molecules, leading to altered cellular activity.

DNA, RNA and genes

DNA is a molecule composed of two chains that coil around each other to form a double helix carrying the genetic instructions used in the growth, development, functioning, and reproduction of all known organisms and many viruses. DNA and ribonucleic acid (RNA) are nucleic acids. Nucleic acids, together with proteins, lipids and complex carbohydrates (polysaccharides), are one of the four major types of macromolecules that are essential for all known forms of life.

The two DNA strands are also known as polynucleotides as they are composed of simpler monomeric units called nucleotides. Each nucleotide is composed of one of four nitrogen-containing nucleobases (cytosine [C], guanine [G], adenine [A] or thymine [T]), a sugar called deoxyribose, and a phosphate group.

Figure 10 is a graphic of DNA replication. The nitrogenous bases of the two separate polynucleotide strands are bound together, according to base pairing rules (A with T and C with G), with hydrogen bonds to make double-stranded DNA in a helical form.

Figure 10. A graphic of DNA replication.

Figure 10.

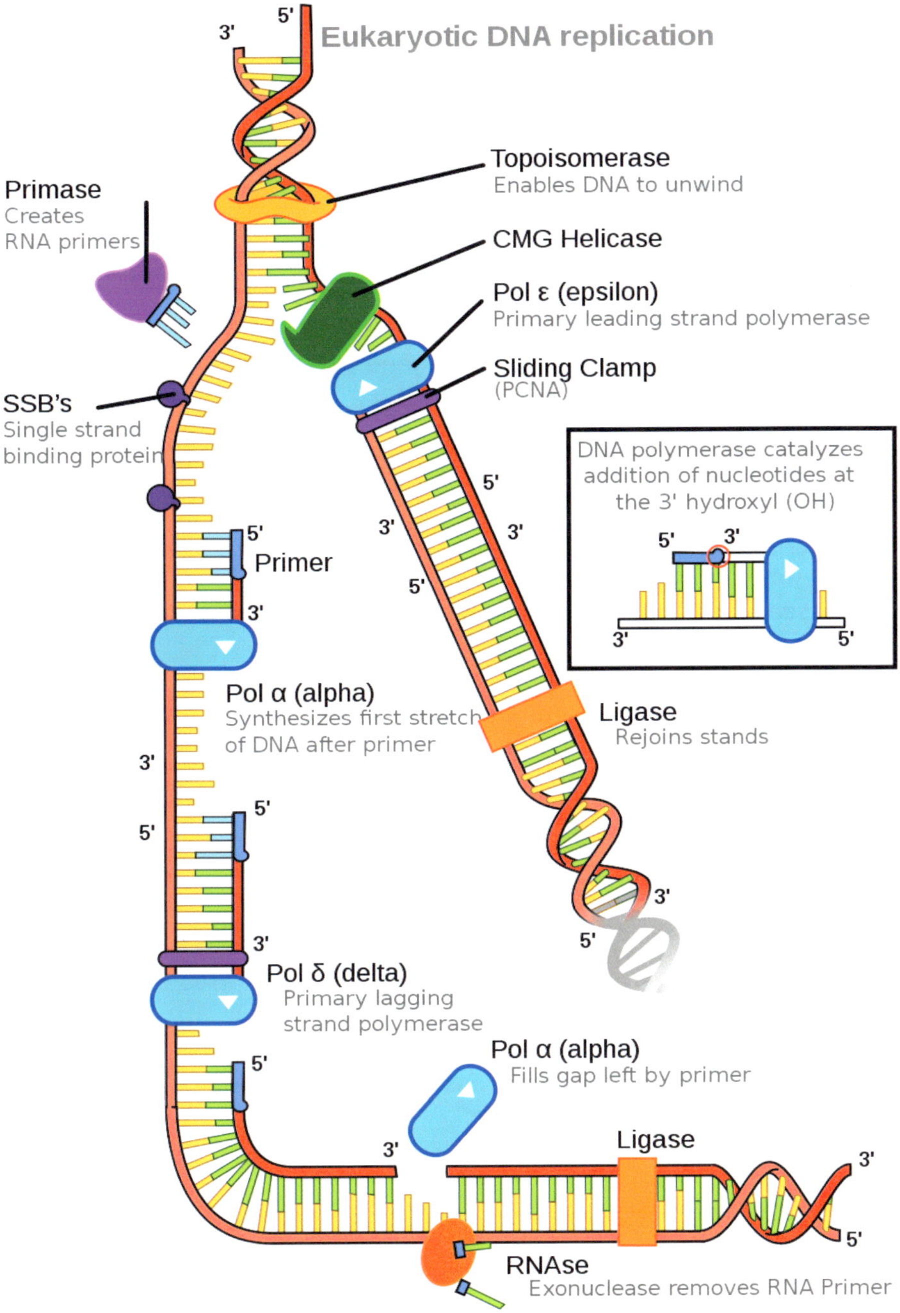

Genes

A gene is a sequence of nucleotides in DNA or RNA that codes for a molecule that has a function. Genes are contained on the chromosomes in the cell nucleus. During gene expression, the DNA is first copied into RNA. The RNA can be directly functional or be the intermediate template for a protein that performs a function. A chromosome consists of a long strand of DNA containing many genes. A human chromosome can have up to 500 million base pairs of DNA with thousands of genes. Gene expression is the process by which information from a gene is used in the synthesis of a functional gene product. These products are often proteins, When the end-product is a protein, genes are first transcribed into RNA, and this transcript is then translated into protein. Several steps in the gene expression process may be modulated, including transcription, RNA splicing, translation and post-translational modification of the protein. Gene regulation gives the cell control over structure and function, and is the basis for cellular differentiation, morphogenesis and the versatility and adaptability of any organism.

Genes are expressed by being transcribed into RNA, and this transcript may then be translated into protein.

Figure 11. Diagram showing how translation of messenger RNA and protein synthesis takes place in ribosomes.

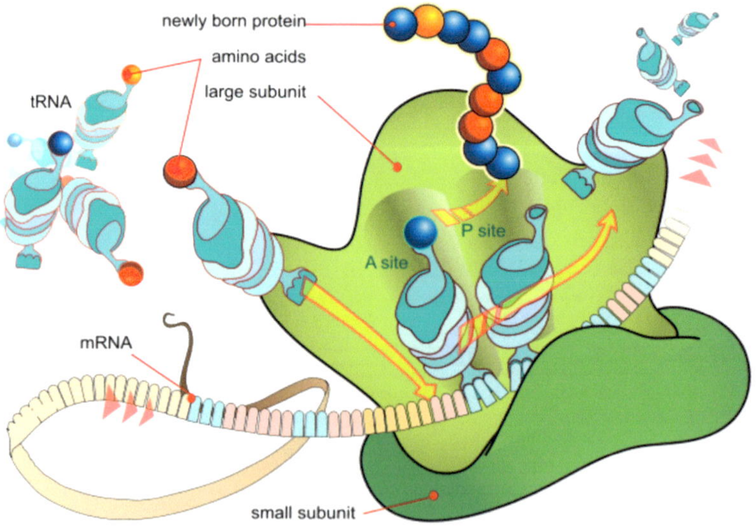

Figure 11. This work has been released into the public domain by its author, LadyofHats. By LadyofHats - Own work based on:[1], [2], [3], [4], [5], [6], [7], and [8]., Public Domain, https://commons.wikimedia.org/w/index.php?curid=4889777;

https://en.wikipedia.org/wiki/Translation_(biology)#/media/File:Ribosome_mRNA_translation_en.svg. No changes have been made to this image.

Protein folding

A polypeptide (protein) folds into its characteristic and functional three-dimensional structure from a random coil. Each protein exists as an unfolded polypeptide or random coil when translated from a sequence of messenger (m) RNA into a linear chain of amino acids (Figure 12, left hand image). Amino acids interact with each other to produce a well-defined three-dimensional structure.

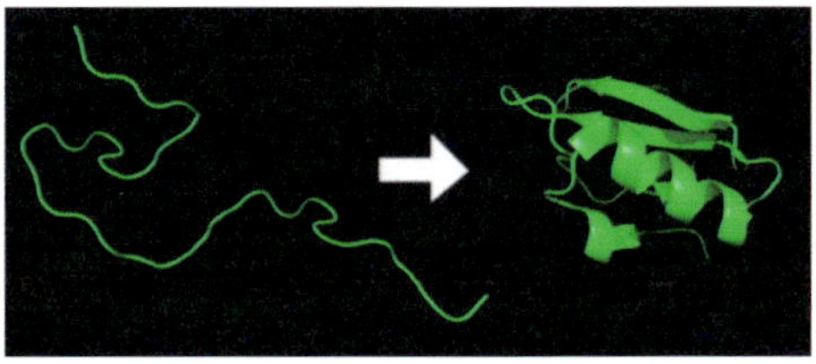

Figure 12 shows a protein before (left) and after (right) folding.

This image, reproduced here from Wikimedia Commons, is in the public domain because its creator has placed it there. By No machine-readable author provided. Dr Kjaergaard assumed (based on copyright claims). - No machine-readable source provided. Own work assumed (based on copyright claims). Public Domain, https://commons.wikimedia.org/w/index.php?curid=1967109. https://en.wikipedia.org/wiki/Protein_folding#/media/File:Protein_folding.png. No changes have been made to this image.

5. The biology of malignant human cells.

Defects in genes (DNA), epigenetic factors and mismatch repair systems can all cause human cells to become malignant.

Genes

With the exception of congenital disorders, malignant human cells have an abnormality of their genetic systems, and differ in this regard to abnormal, but non-malignant, as well as to normal human cells. Carcinogenesis is the formation of a cancer, whereby normal cells are transformed into cancer cells. The process is characterized by changes at the cellular, genetic, and epigenetic levels and abnormal cell division. Cell division is a physiological process that occurs in almost all tissues and under a variety of circumstances. Normally the balance between proliferation and programmed cell death, in the form of apoptosis, is maintained to ensure the integrity of tissues and organs. According to the prevailing accepted theory of carcinogenesis, the somatic mutation

theory, mutations in DNA and epimutations that lead to cancer disrupt these orderly processes by disrupting the programming regulating the processes, upsetting the normal balance between proliferation and cell death. This results in uncontrolled cell division and the evolution of those cells by natural selection in the body. Only certain mutations lead to cancer whereas the majority of mutations do not.

A series of several mutations to certain classes of genes is usually required before a normal cell will transform into a malignant cell.

In order for a normal cell to transform into a malignant cell, the genes that regulate cell growth and differentiation must be altered.

The affected genes are divided into two broad categories. Oncogenes are genes that promote cell growth and reproduction. Tumor suppressor genes are genes that inhibit cell division and survival. Malignant transformation can occur through the formation of novel oncogenes, the inappropriate over-expression of normal oncogenes, or by the under-expression or disabling of tumor suppressor genes. Typically, changes in multiple genes are required to transform a normal cell into a cancer cell (Figure 13)

Figure 13 illustrates that cancers are caused by a series of mutations. Each mutation alters the behavior of the cell to some extent.

Figure 13.

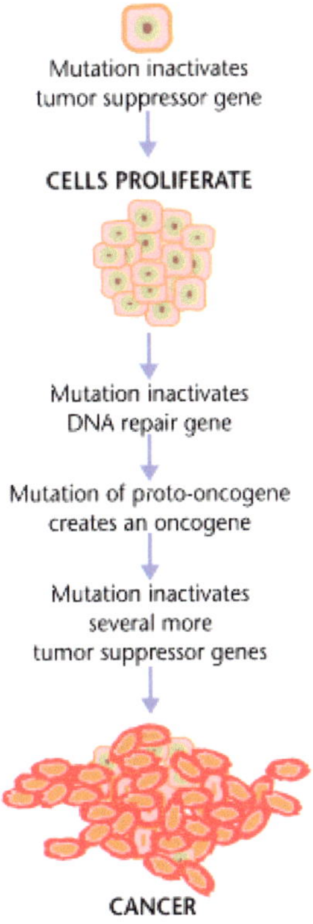

The abnormal biological properties of human malignant cells can be summarized as follows:

- Acquisition of self-sufficiency in growth signals, leading to unchecked growth.
- Loss of sensitivity to anti-growth signals, also leading to unchecked growth.
- Loss of capacity for apoptosis, allowing growth despite genetic errors and external anti-growth signals.

- Loss of capacity for senescence, leading to limitless replicative potential (immortality).
- Acquisition of sustained angiogenesis, allowing the tumor to grow beyond the limitations of passive nutrient diffusion.
- Acquisition of ability to invade neighbouring tissues, the defining property of invasive carcinoma.
- Acquisition of ability to seed metastases at distant sites, a late-appearing property of some malignant tumors (carcinomas or others).

Involved in these steps is

- Loss of capacity to repair genetic errors, leading to an increased mutation rate (genomic instability), thus accelerating all the above changes.

Often, the multiple genetic changes that result in cancer may take many years to accumulate. During this time, the biological behavior of the pre-malignant cells slowly changes from the properties of normal cells to those with cancer-like properties (Figure 14).

Figure 14. Figure 14 shows that tissue can be organized in a continuous spectrum from normal to malignant.

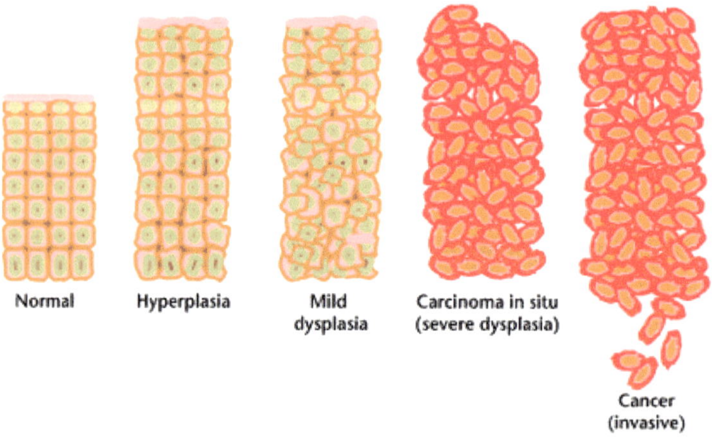

This image, reproduced here from Wikimedia Commons, is in the public domain because it is a work prepared by an officer or employee of the United States Government as part of that person's official duties under the terms of Title 17, Chapter 1, Section 105 of the US Code. By Unknown author - National Cancer Institute (archived), Public Domain, https://commons.wikimedia.org/w/index.php?curid=658483. No changes have been made to this image.

Epigenetic factors also plays a major role in the development of human cancers.

Epigenetic modifications to the DNA of cancer cells do not involve a change in the nucleotide sequence, but instead involve a change in the way the genetic code is expressed. Epigenetic alterations may be just as important, or even more important, than genetic mutations in a cell's transformation to malignancy. In malignant cells loss of expression of genes occurs about 10 times more frequently by transcription silencing (caused by epigenetic promoter hypermethylation of CpG islands) than by mutations. In different types of cancer, a variety of epigenetic mechanisms can be perturbed, such as silencing of tumor suppressor genes and activation of oncogenes by altered CpG island methylation patterns, histone modifications, and dysregulation of DNA-binding proteins (Figure 15)

Figure 15. This figure shows epigenetic patterns in a normal and cancer cells.

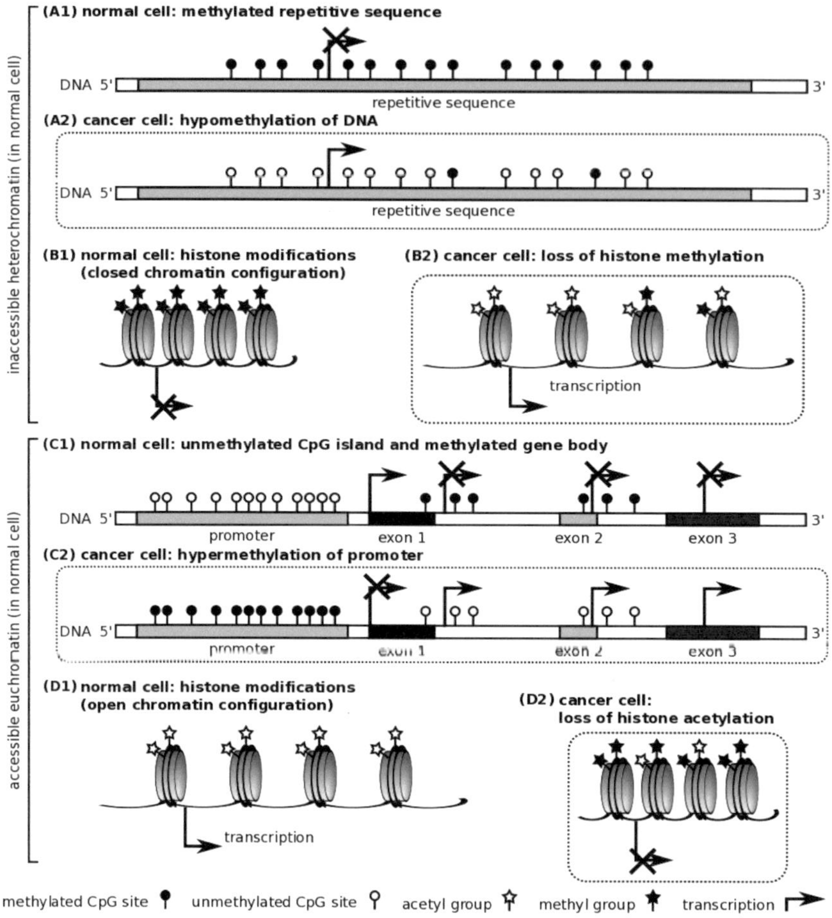

Figure 16 shows a DNA molecule that is methylated on both strands on the center cytosine. DNA methylation plays an important role for epigenetic gene regulation in development and cancer. The image shows the crystal structure of a short DNA helix with sequence "accgcCGgcgcc", which is methylated on both strands at the center cytosine.

https://commons.wikimedia.org/w/index.php?curid=17066877. The structure was taken from the Protein Data Bank (accession number 329D), rendering was performed with VMD (Visual Molecular Dynamics rendering program) and post-processing was done in Photoshop]. No change has been made to this image.

Figure 16. A DNA molecule that is methylated on both strands on the center cytosine.

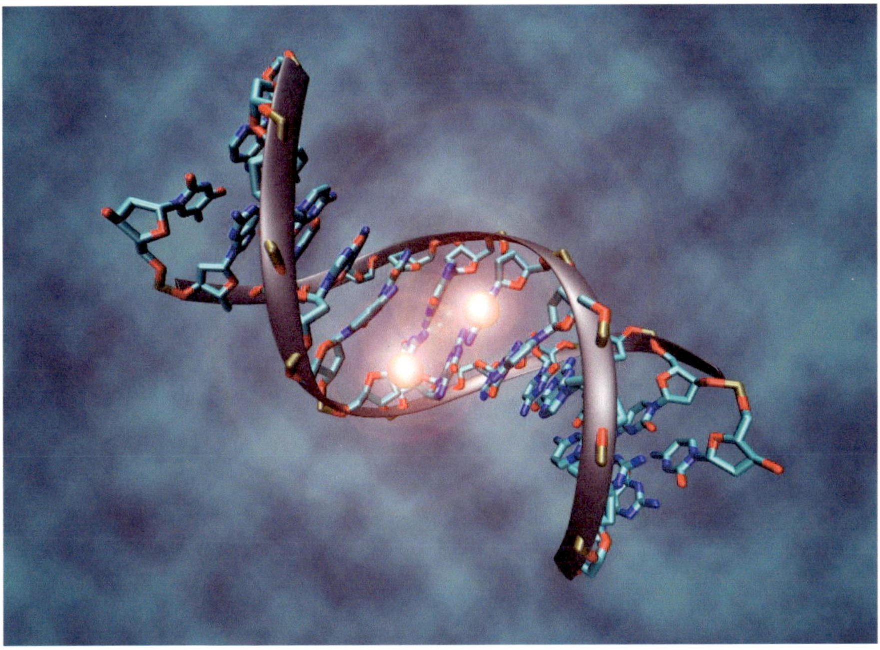

DNA mismatch repair systems

If DNA repair is deficient, DNA damage tends to accumulate. Such excess DNA damage can increase mutational errors during DNA replication. Excess DNA damage can also increase epigenetic alterations due to errors during DNA repair. Such mutations and epigenetic alterations can give rise to malignancy. Germ line mutations in DNA repair genes cause only 2–5% of colon cancer cases. However, altered expression of microRNAs, causing DNA repair deficiencies, are frequently associated with cancers and may be an important causal factor for such cancers.

In non-hereditary cancers, a deficiency in DNA repair is occasionally found to be due to a mutation in a DNA repair gene, but reduced or absent expression of DNA repair genes is much more frequently due to epigenetic alterations that reduce or silence gene expression.

Cancer therapy procedures such as chemotherapy and radiotherapy work by overwhelming the capacity of the malignant cells to repair DNA damage, resulting in their death. Cells that are most rapidly dividing – most typically cancer cells – are preferentially affected. An important side-effect is that other non-cancerous but rapidly dividing cells such as progenitor cells in the gut, skin, and hematopoietic system are also affected. Modern cancer treatments attempt to localize the DNA damage to cells and tissues only associated with cancer, either by physical means (concentrating the therapeutic agent in the region of the tumor) or by biochemical means (exploiting a feature unique to cancer cells in the body).

5. Clinical and pathological features of non-melanoma skin cancers

5.1. Cutaneous squamous cell carcinoma

Cutaneous squamous-cell carcinoma (cSCC) usually presents as a hard lump with a scaly top but can also form an ulcer (Figures 17 - 19).

Figure 17. Cutaneous squamous cell carcinoma on the nose. CSCCs tend to arise from pre-malignant lesions such as actinic keratoses; the surface is usually scaly and often ulcerates (as shown here). This image is by Unknown photographer/artist - http://visualsonline.cancer.gov/details.cfm?imageid=2165, Public Domain, https://commons.wikimedia.org/w/index.php?curid=859316. https://en.wikipedia.org/wiki/Squamous_cell_skin_cancer#/media/File:Squamous_Cell_Carcinoma.jpg This work is in the public domain in the United States because it is a work prepared by an officer or employee of the United States Government as part of that person's official duties under the terms of Title 17, Chapter 1, Section 105 of the US Code. No changes have been made to this image.

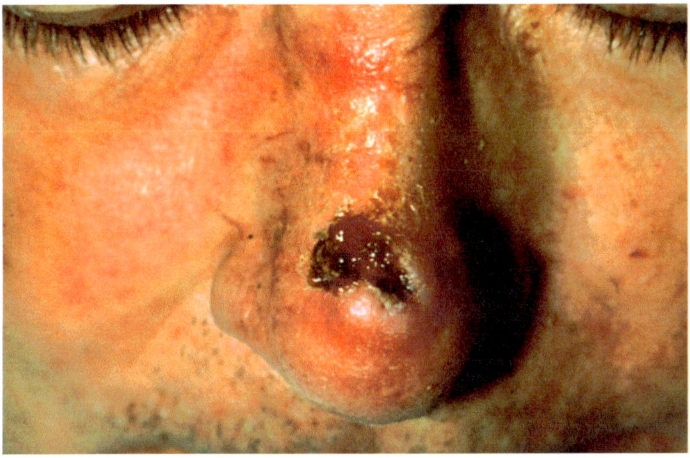

Figure 18. Cutaneous squamous cell carcinoma on the dorsum of the hand.

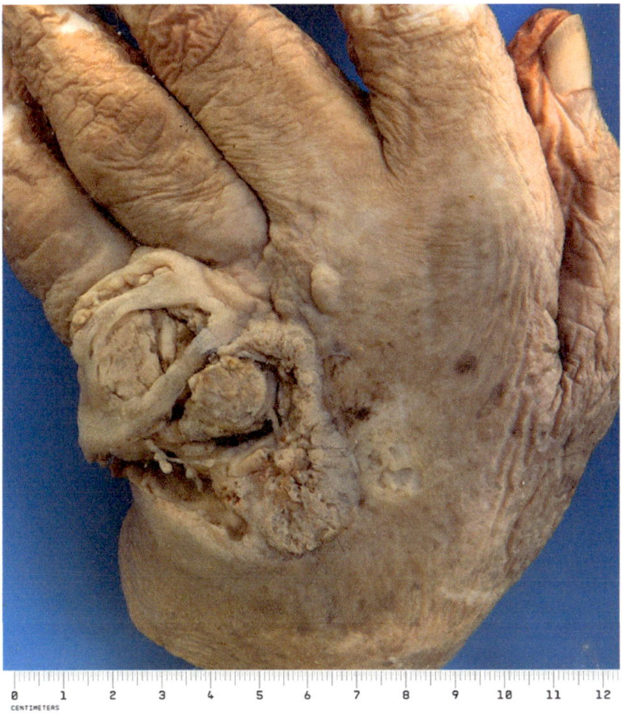

.

This 64 year old man had 5 years previously noticed a small lump on the dorsum of his left hand. This had gradually increased in size over 2 years; it had become painful and the skin started to ulcerate over it. He refused local resection at this stage. The lesion progressed to an enormous ulcer with severe pain, and infiltration and involvement of tendons and nerves of the medial three fingers. He underwent amputation of the forearm 2 inches below the elbow.

This image is by the University of Cape Town Pathology Learning Centre: Jurgen Geitner - https://digitalpathology.uct.ac.za/case_detail.php?case_id=4227, CC BY-SA 4.0, https://commons.wikimedia.org/w/index.php?curid=82553112. https://en.wikipedia.org/wiki/Squamous_cell_skin_cancer#/media/File:Squamous-carcinoma-of-dorsum-of-hand.jpg. This file is licensed under the Creative Commons Attribution-Share Alike 4.0 International license. No changes have been made to this image.

Figure 19. Gross slice of a resected squamous cell carcinoma of the skin.

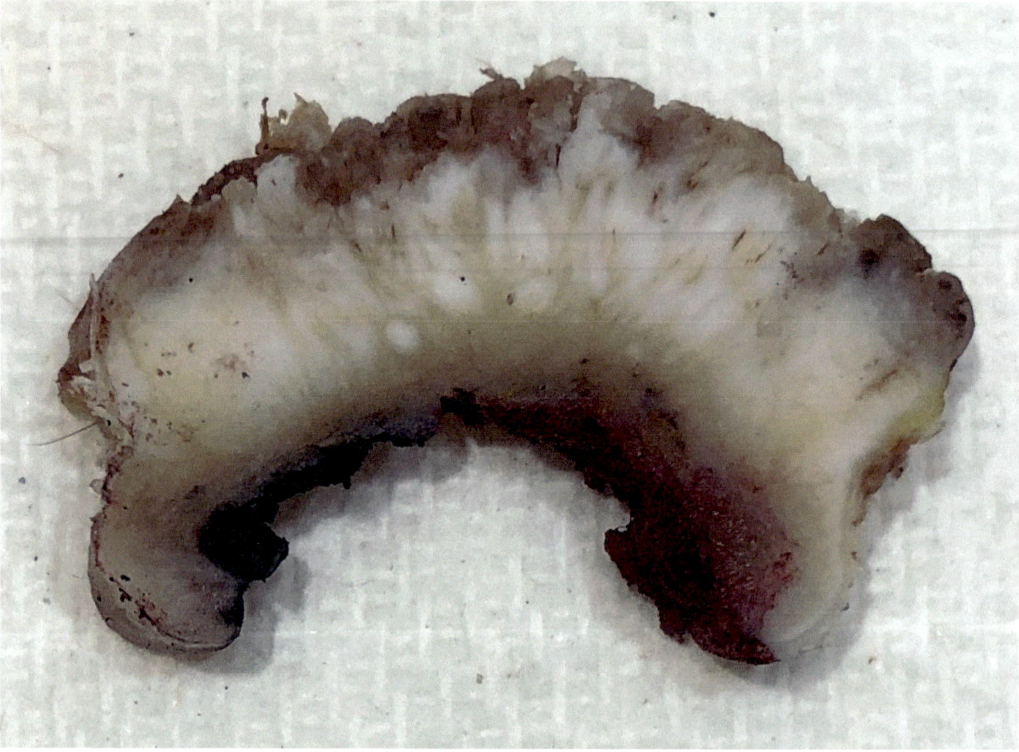

This image is by Mikael Häggström, M.D.- Author info- Reusing images- Conflicts of interest: NoneMikael HäggströmConsent note: Consent from the patient or patient's relatives is regarded as redundant, because of absence of identifiable features (List of HIPAA identifiers) in the media and case information (See also HIPAA case reports guidance). - Own work, CC0, https://commons.wikimedia.org/w/index.php?curid=96668633. https://en.wikipedia.org/wiki/Squamous_cell_skin_cancer#/media/File:Gross_pathology_of_squamous_cell_carcinoma.jpg. This file is made available under the Creative Commons CC0 1.0 Universal Public Domain Dedication. No changes have been made to this image.

Figure 20. Histopathology of cutaneous squamous cell carcinoma. Well-differentiated (and yet invasive) cSCC, showing prominent keratinization and sometimes form "pearl-like" structures where dermal nests of keratinocytes attempt to mature in a layered fashion. Well-differentiated SCC has slightly enlarged, hyperchromatic nuclei with abundant amounts of cytoplasm. Intercellular bridges will frequently be visible.

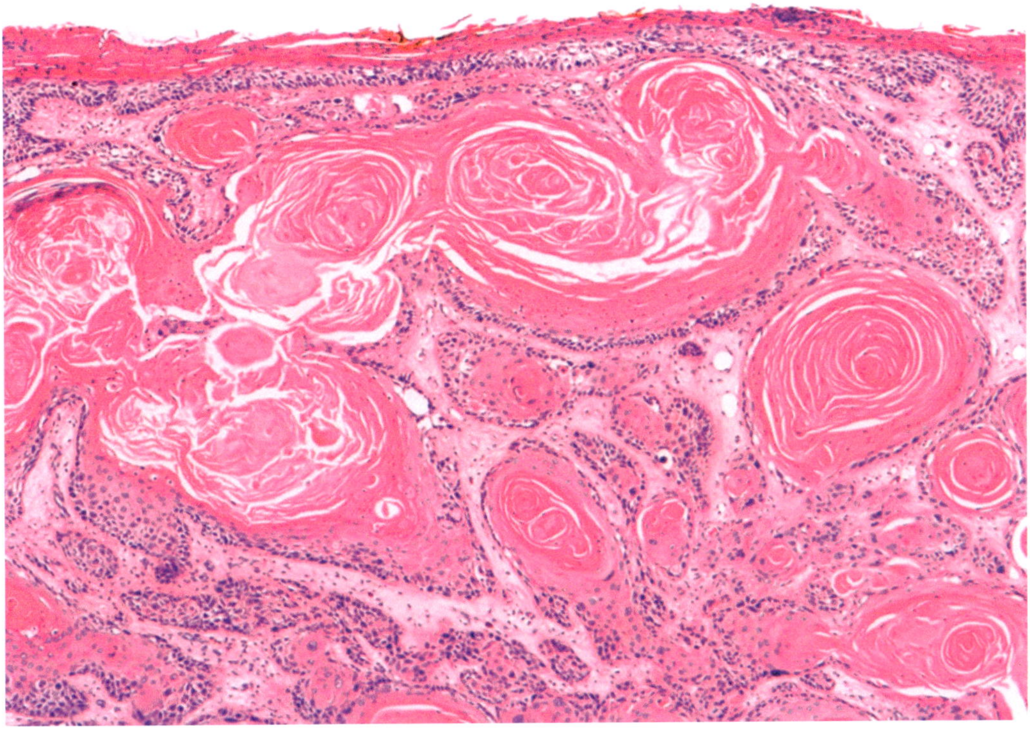

Cutaneous SCC cancer is much more likely to spread to distant areas than basal cell cancer.

The main risk factor is high total exposure to ultraviolet radiation from the sun, and for this reason the highest global incidence is among fair-skinned people in Australia (Figure 21).

Figure 21. Age-standardized death from melanoma and other skin cancers per 100,000 inhabitants in 2004. no data less than 0.7 0.7–1.4 1.4–2.1 2.1–2.8 2.8–3.5 3.5–4.2 4.2–4.9 4.9–5.6 5.6–6.3 6.3–7 7–7.7 more than 7.7.

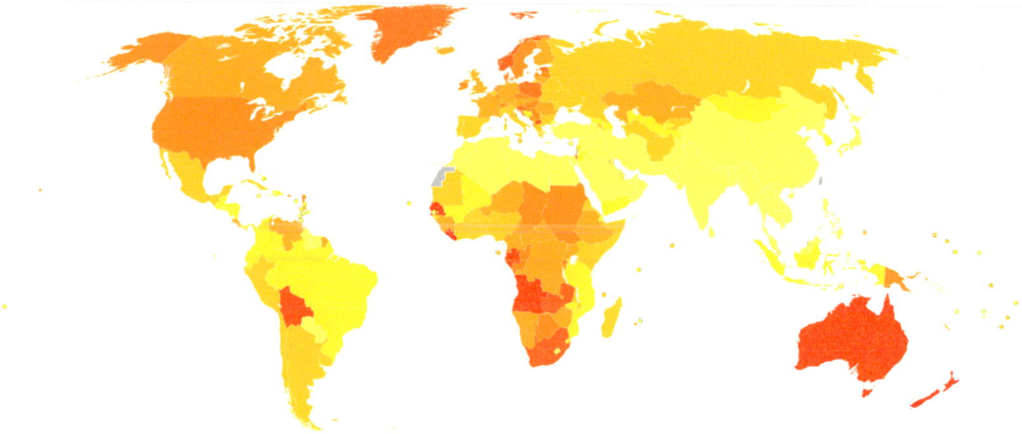

Thus, SCCs usually occur in areas of the body commonly exposed to the sun; the face, ears, neck, hands, or arm. People who have had an SCC due to sun damage to their skin are more likely to develop further SCCs or melanomas and, after initial treatment has been completed, such individuals should have a skin surveillance examination by a dermatologist every four months long-term.

Another risk factor is immunosuppression. This is most commonly seen in people who have received an organ transplant and who are on long-term immunosuppressive medication to prevent rejection of the transplanted organ. While the risk of developing all skin cancers increases with these medications, this effect is particularly severe for SCC, with hazard ratios as high as 250 being reported, versus 40 for basal cell carcinoma. The incidence of SCC development increases with time posttransplant. Heart and lung transplant recipients are at the highest risk of developing SCC. The risk of SCC, and non-melanoma skin cancers generally, varies with the immunosuppressive drug regimen chosen. The risk is greatest with calcineurin inhibitors such as cyclosporine and tacrolimus, and least with m-TOR inhibitors, such as sirolimus and everolimus. The antimetabolites azathioprine and mycophenolic acid have an intermediate risk profile.

Risk is also elevated in certain genetic skin disorders, such as xeroderma pigmentosum and some forms of epidermolysis bullosa.

Diagnosis should be confirmed by tissue biopsy (Figure 20).

Treatment is usually by surgical removal. This can be by simple excision if the cancer is small, otherwise Mohs surgery is generally recommended.

In the cases in which distant spread has occurred chemotherapy or biologic or specifically designed therapy may be used: targeted therapeutic agents that have been approved for therapeutic use by the USA Food and Drug Administration (FDA) are detailed later in this book.

Cutaneous SCC cancer is much more likely to spread to distant areas than basal cell cancer. If metastatic spread occurs, the five-year survival is approximately 34%. In 2015 it resulted in about 51,900 deaths globally. The usual age at diagnosis is around 66.

The pathological appearance of a squamous cell cancer varies with the depth of the biopsy. For that reason, a biopsy including the subcutaneous tissue and basilar epithelium, to the surface is necessary for correct diagnosis. The performance of a shave biopsy might not acquire enough information for a diagnosis. An inadequate biopsy might be read as actinic keratosis with follicular involvement. A deeper biopsy down to the dermis or subcutaneous tissue might reveal the true status of the cancer.

In invasive SCC, tumor cells infiltrate through the basement membrane. The infiltrate can be somewhat difficult to detect in the early stages of invasion: however, additional indicators such as full thickness epidermal atypia and the involvement of hair follicles can be used to facilitate the diagnosis. Later stages of invasion are characterized by the formation of nests of atypical tumor cells in the dermis, often with a corresponding inflammatory infiltrate.

Surgical block dissection is used if involved regional lymph nodes are present.

5.2. Basal cell carcinoma of the skin

Basal-cell carcinoma (BCC), also known as basal-cell cancer or “rodent ulcer”, is the most common type of skin cancer. It often appears as a painless raised area of skin, which may be shiny with small blood vessels running over it. It may also present as a raised area with ulceration. Basal-cell cancer grows slowly and can damage the tissue around it, but it is unlikely to spread to distant areas or result in death.

Figure 21. Basal cell carcinoma in a 75 year old man.

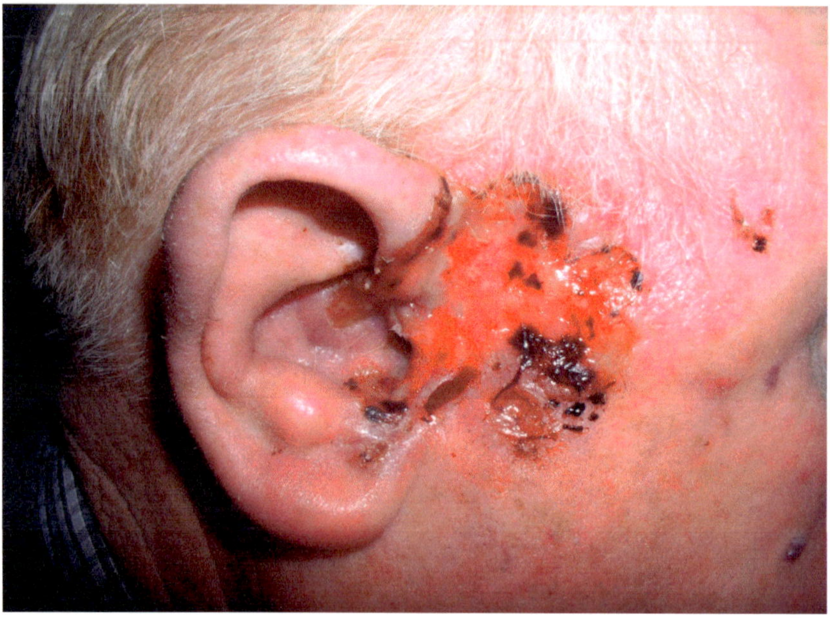

Figure 22. Photograph of a basal cell carcinoma showing telangiectatic blood vessels in the tumor.

Figure 22.

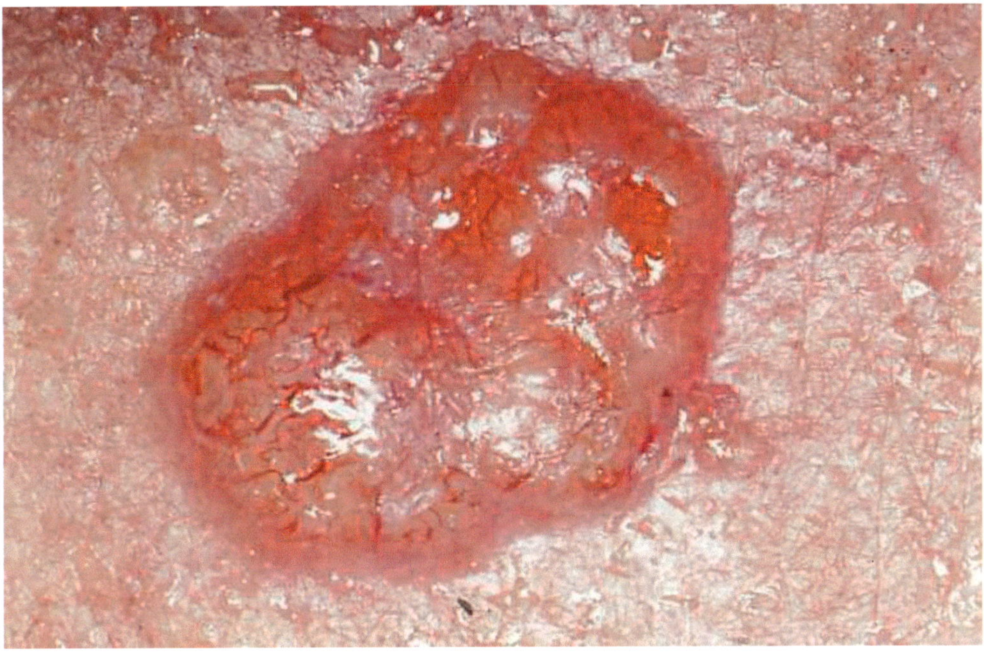

This image is by No machine-readable author provided. John Hendrix assumed (based on copyright claims). - No machine-readable source provided. Own work assumed (based on copyright claims)., Public Domain, https://commons.wikimedia.org/w/index.php?curid=1216868. https://en.wikipedia.org/wiki/Basal-cell_carcinoma#/media/File:Basal_cell_carcinoma.jpg. the copyright holder of this work, release this work into the public domain. This applies worldwide. The author is John Hendrix assumed (based on copyright claims). No changes have been made to this image.

Figure 23. Basal cell carcinoma just below the lower eyelid.

This image is by SkarmoutsosV - Own work, CC BY-SA 4.0, https://commons.wikimedia.org/w/index.php?curid=59759446. https://en.wikipedia.org/wiki/Basal-cell_carcinoma#/media/File:Basal-cell_Carcinoma.jpg. This file is licensed under the Creative Commons Attribution-Share Alike 4.0 International license. No changes have been made to this image.

Figure 23. Basal cell carcinoma just below the nostril.

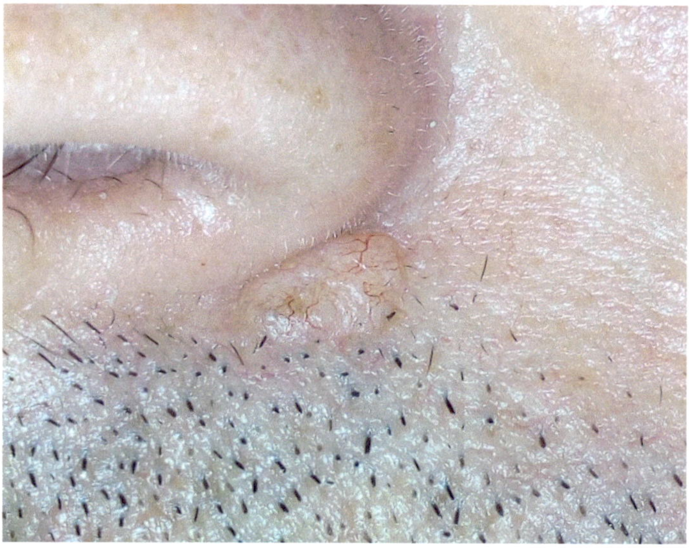

Figure 24. Basal cell carcinoma involving the nose in an elderly man.

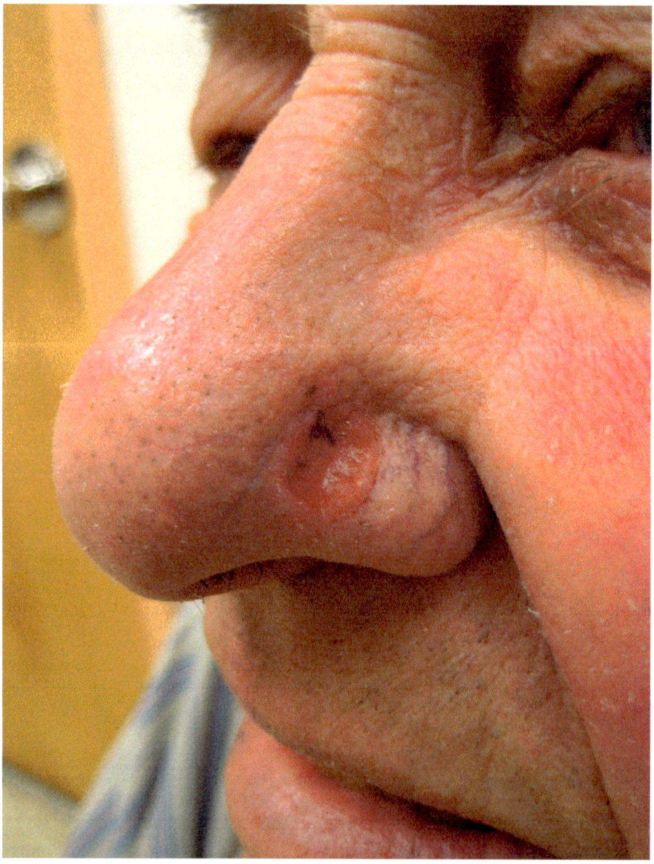

This image is by By James Heilman, MD - Own work, CC BY 3.0, https://commons.wikimedia.org/w/index.php?curid=6827823. https://en.wikipedia.org/wiki/Basal-cell_carcinoma#/media/File:Basal_cell_carcinoma2.JPG. This file is licensed under the Creative Commons Attribution 3.0 Unported license. The uploader asserts the following regarding consent of identifiable persons:

I (James Heilman) personally created this media. All identifiable persons shown specifically consented to publication of this photograph. No changes have been made to this image.

The diagnosis should be made on histopathology of the lesion (Figure 25, 26)

Figure 25. Micrograph of a basal-cell carcinoma, showing the characteristic histomorphologic features (peripheral palisading, myxoid stroma, artefactual clefting). H&E stain.

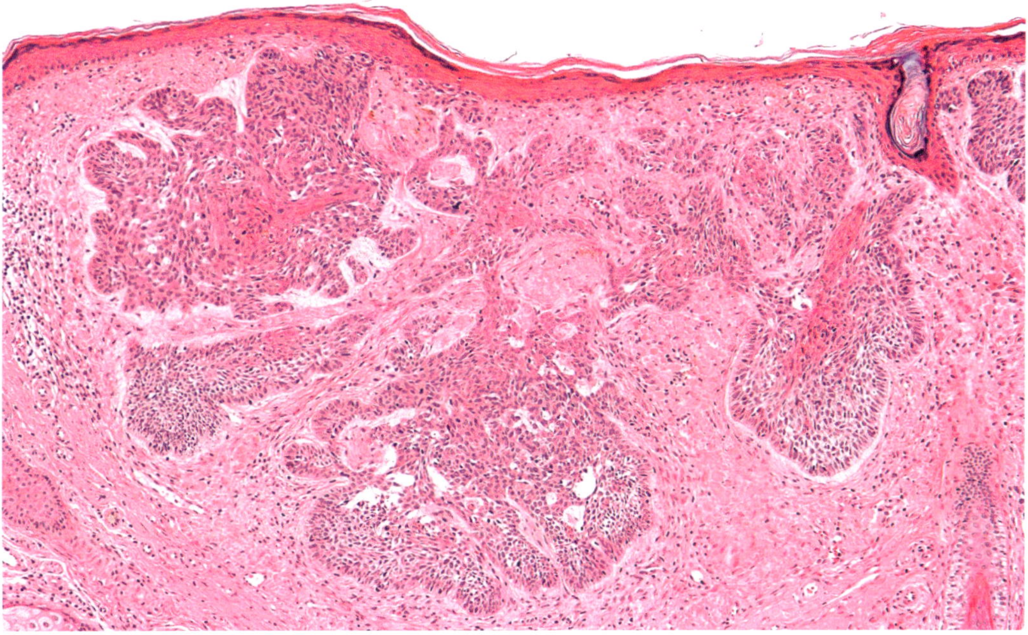

This image is by Nephron - Own work, CC BY-SA 3.0, https://commons.wikimedia.org/w/index.php?curid=22082605. https://en.wikipedia.org/wiki/Basal-cell_carcinoma#/media/File:Basal_cell_carcinoma_-_2_-_intermed_mag.jpg. This file is licensed under the Creative Commons Attribution-Share Alike 3.0 Unported license. No changes have been made to this image.

Figure 26. Comparison H&E stain (left) with BerEP4 immunohistochemistry staining (right) on a pathological section having BCC with squamous cell metaplasia. Only BCC cells are stained with BerEP4. (100x magnification)

Figure 26.

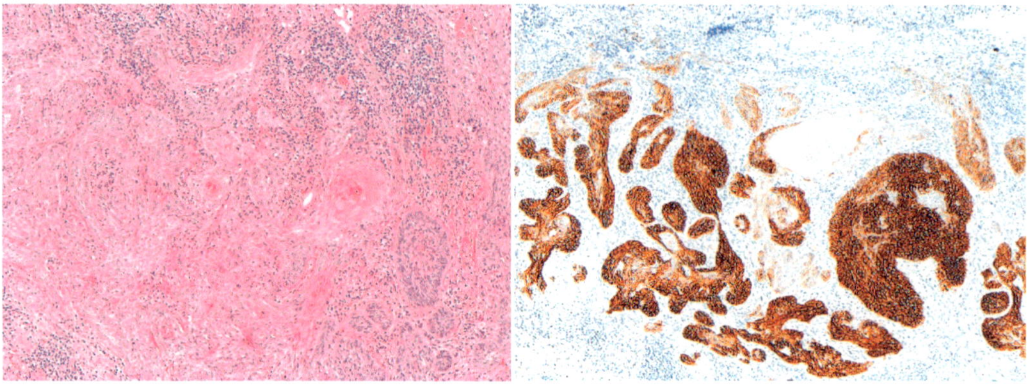

Risk factors include exposure to ultraviolet light, having lighter skin, radiation therapy, long-term exposure to arsenic and poor immune-system function. Exposure to UV light during childhood is particularly harmful. Tanning beds have become another common source of ultraviolet radiation. Diagnosis usually depends on skin examination, confirmed by tissue biopsy.

Treatment is typically by surgical removal. This can be by simple excision if the cancer is small; otherwise, Mohs surgery is generally recommended. Radiotherapy is generally used in older patients who are not candidates for surgery. It is also used in cases where surgical excision will be disfiguring or difficult to reconstruct (especially on the tip of the nose, and the nostril rims). Radiation treatment with external radiation often takes as few as 5 visits to as many as 25 visits. Usually, the more visits scheduled for therapy, the less complication or damage is done to the normal tissue supporting the tumor. Radiotherapy can also be useful if surgical excision has been done incompletely or if the pathology report following surgery suggests a high risk of recurrence, for example if nerve involvement has been demonstrated. Cure rate can be as high as 95% for small tumor, or as low as 80% for large tumors. In the rare cases in which distant spread has occurred, chemotherapy or targeted therapy may be used.

Recently, two drugs – sonidegib and vismodegib that specifically target the Hedgehog intracellular signalling system, have been approved for use in basal cell carcinoma and are described in detail in Section 8 of this book

Pathogenesis

A mutation in the SMO (smoothed) gene, which is in the Hedgehog intracellular signalling pathway causes basal cell carcinoma, and two drugs (vismodegib and sonidegib) targeting this abnormality have been specifically designed to disrupt this pathway (see Section 8)

Prognosis

The prognosis is excellent if the appropriate method of treatment is used in early primary basal-cell cancers. Recurrent cancers are much harder to cure, with a higher recurrent rate with any methods of treatment. Although basal-cell carcinoma rarely metastasizes, it grows locally with invasion and destruction of local tissues. The cancer can impinge on vital structures like nerves and result in loss of sensation or loss of function or rarely death. The vast majority of cases can be successfully treated before serious complications occur.

5.3. Merkel cell carcinoma[a]

Merkel cell carcinoma (MCC) is a rare and aggressive skin cancer occurring in about 3 people per 1,000,000 members of the population. It is also known as cutaneous APUDoma, primary neuroendocrine carcinoma of the skin, primary small cell carcinoma of the skin, and trabecular carcinoma of the skin. Factors involved in the development of MCC include the Merkel cell polyomavirus (MCPyV or MCV), a weakened immune system, and exposure to ultraviolet radiation. Merkel-cell carcinoma usually arises on the head, neck, and extremities, as well as in the perianal region and on the eyelid. It is more common in people over 60 years of age, Caucasian people, and males. MCC is less common in children.

Merkel cell carcinoma (MCC) usually presents as a firm nodule (up to 2 cm diameter) or mass (>2 cm diameter). These flesh-colored, red, or blue tumors typically vary in size from 0.5 cm (less than one-quarter of an inch) to more than 5 cm (2 inches) in diameter and may enlarge rapidly. Tumors can present as painless, tender or itchy, and other MCC manifestations as papules or plaques have also been reported.

Figure 27. The small spot on the left arm is Merkel cell carcinoma.

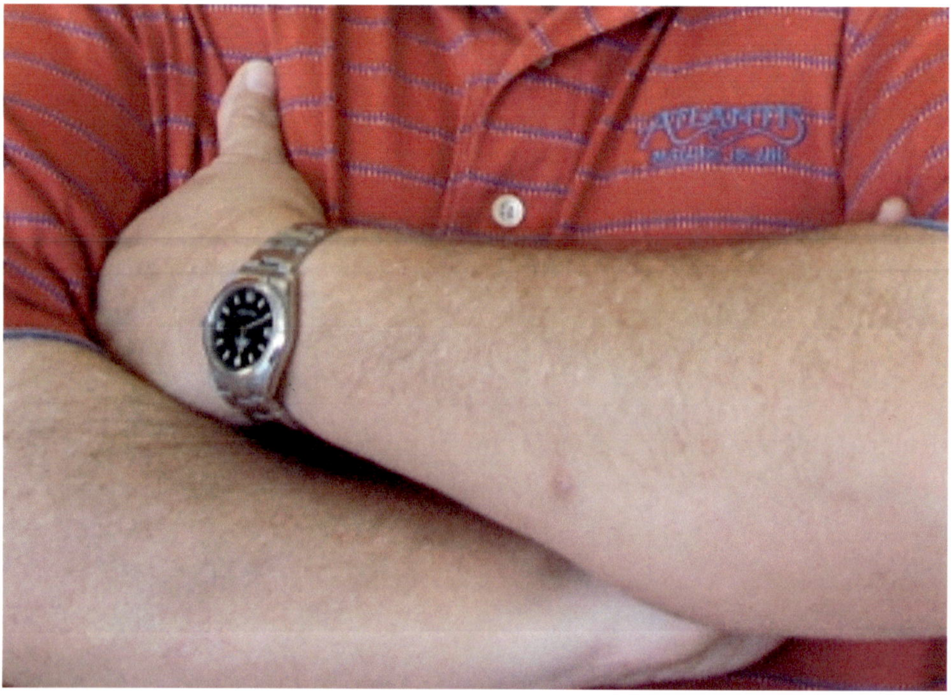

This image is by George from Charleston, AmeriKa - Smallest Bump On Arm Is Cancer, CC BY 2.0, https://commons.wikimedia.org/w/index.php?curid=5783923. https://en.wikipedia.org/wiki/Merkel-cell_carcinoma#/media/File:Merkel_cell_carcinoma_arm.jpg. This file is licensed under the Creative Commons Attribution 2.0 Generic license. No changes have been made to this image.

Figure 28. Resected specimen of Merkel cell carcinoma. This large tumor presented as a protuberant mass on the buttock of a 45-year-old woman. Microscopically it showed sheets of undifferentiated cells with high nuclear/cytoplasmic ratio, a high mitotic rate, and an occasional inconspicuous nucleoli. Immunostaining showed strong dot-like and diffuse cytoplasmic positivity for cytokeratin 20, CAM5.2, and

AE1-AE3, as well as granular staining for synaptophysin and chromogranin. There were negative reactions for cytokeratin 7, gross cystic disease fluid protein 15, melan-A, S-100 protein, and thyroid transcription factor 1-alpha.

Even though the histologic features and immunostain profile was characteristic of a primary skin tumor, the presentation is atypical. Usually, Merkel cell carcinoma presents on the sun-exposed areas of elderly individuals. Therefore, the pathologist recommended workup for the possibility of another primary site, including lung, female genital tract, salivary gland, and other cutaneous site.

Figure 28. Resected Merkel cell carcinoma of the skin

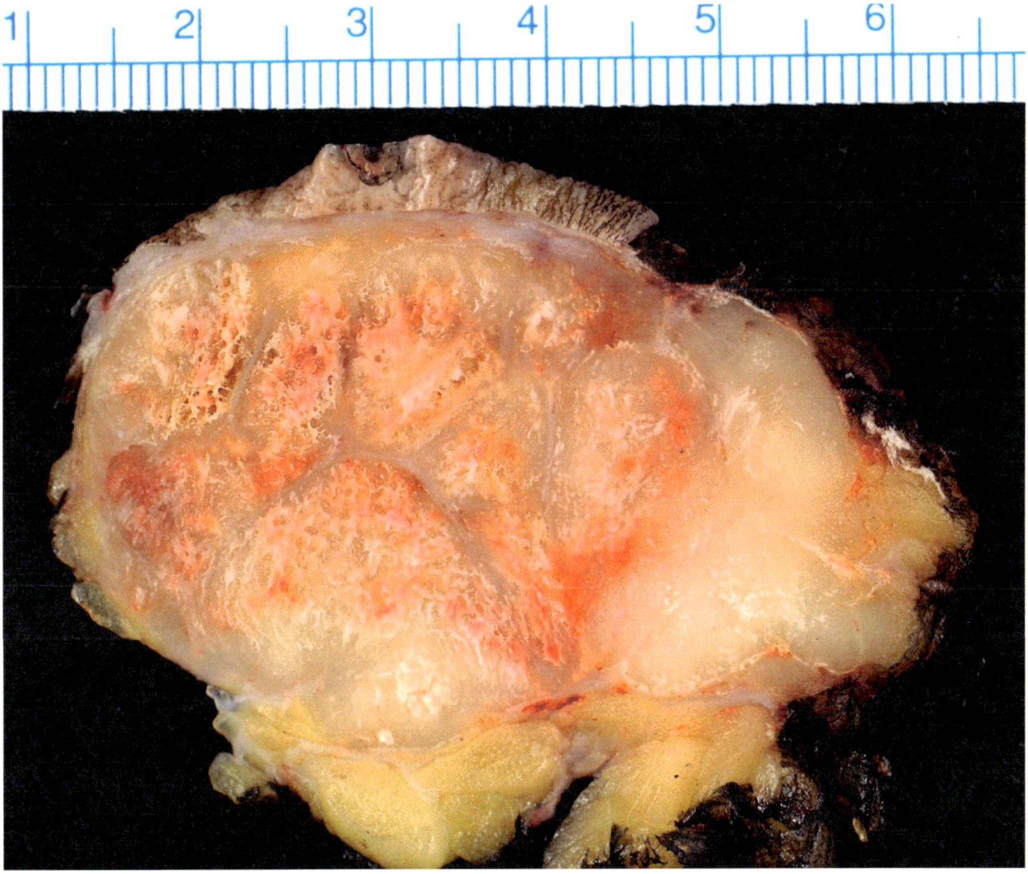

This image is by Ed Uthman from Houston, TX, USA - Merkel Cell Carcinoma, CC BY-SA 2.0, https://commons.wikimedia.org/w/index.php?curid=3852062. https://en.wikipedia.org/wiki/Merkel-cell_carcinoma#/media/File:Merkel_Cell_Carcinoma_buttock_45-year-old_woman.jpg. This file is licensed under the Creative Commons Attribution-Share Alike 2.0 Generic license. No changes were made to this image.

MCC is sometimes mistaken for other histological types of cancer, including basal cell carcinoma, cutaneous squamous cell carcinoma, malignant melanoma, lymphoma, and small cell carcinoma, or as a benign cyst.

Merkel cell cancers tend to invade locally, infiltrating the underlying subcutaneous fat, fascia, and muscle, and typically metastasize early in their natural history, most often to the regional lymph nodes. MCCs can also spread aggressively through the blood vessels to many organs, particularly to liver, lung, brain, and bone.

Diagnosis is made by histopathological examination of the resected lesion, including immunostaining (Figure 29).

Figure 29. Photomicrographs of a typical Merkel cell carcinoma.

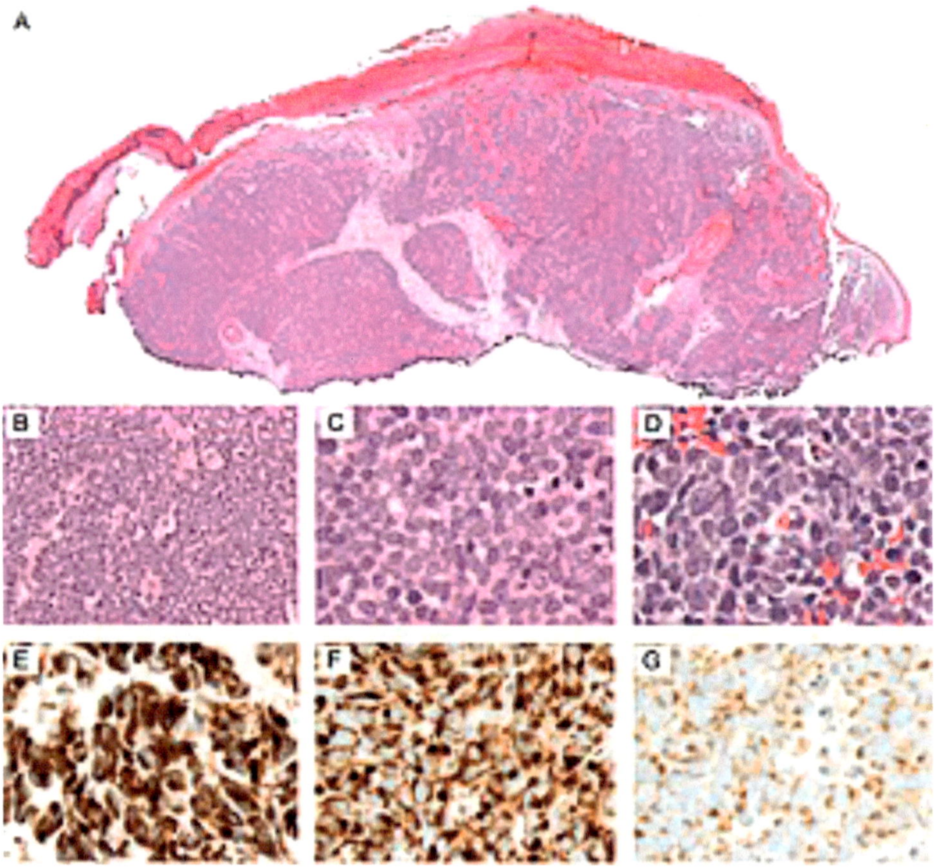

Photomicrographs of a typical Merkel-cell carcinoma at A) 4, B) 40x, and C–D) 100x objectives. Hematoxylin and eosin staining demonstrates small, undifferentiated cells with high N/C ratio and scanty cytoplasm. The typical immunopanel demonstrates positive staining with E) cytokeratin AE1/AE3 (100x oil immersion); F) CK 20 (100x oil immersion), and neuroendocrine markers such as G) chromogranin (100x oil immersion).

MCC is rare, and expedient referral to a radiation oncologist is critical. MCC will quickly relapse following any attempted excisional biopsy. Radiation therapy is the primary management of Merkel cell carcinoma. The largest series are from Australia and have demonstrated that radiotherapy alone achieves equal outcomes with upfront or neoadjuvant surgery followed by radiation therapy. The role of surgery is now to perform a biopsy. There have been no head-to-head trials comparing the two treatment strategies, and in the absence of this, surgeons tend to most commonly perform excisional biopsy prior to referring for radiation therapy. MCC is exquisitely radiosensitive.

There is currently no role for chemotherapy in this disease.

Immunotherapies, namely inhibitors of the PD1-PDL1 checkpoint signalling pathway, are novel anticancer agents that have shown benefit in advanced-stage MCC. The PD-1 pathway is responsible for regulating the balance between T-cell activation and over-activation leading to T-cell exhaustion or autoimmunity.

PD1/PDL1 pathway inhibitors approved or in clinical trials for use in MCC treatment include:

Avelumab to treat adults and children above 12 years with metastatic MCC.

Pembrolisumab for all ages (adults and pediatrics) with recurrent locally advanced or metastatic Merkel cell carcinoma.

Other PD1/PD1L checkpoint inhibitors are in clinical trials for MCC

Prognosis

According to the American Joint Committee on Cancer (AJCC), the natural course of MCC is "variable and depends heavily on the stage at diagnosis". Staging of MCC is classified according to the TNM staging system, a notation system that describes the stage of cancer according to the size of the primary tumor (T), the degree of spread to regional lymph nodes (N), and the presence of distant metastasis (M). A combination of T, N, and M stages dictate the final clinical stage group (0, I, IIA, IIB, IIIA, IIIB, IV).[45] Advanced stage (i.e. increased size of the tumor, spreading of the tumor into surrounding and/or distant tissue, and involvement of lymph nodes) is associated with lower survival rates.

The National Cancer Data Base has survival rates collected from nearly 3000 MCC patients from year 1996–2000 with 5-year survival rates listed as follows: Stage IA: 80%. Stage IB: 60%. Stage IIA: 60%. Stage IIB: 50%. Stage IIC: 50%. Stage IIIA: 45%. Stage IIIB: 25%. Stage IV: 20%. 5 yr survival may be 51% among people with localized disease, 35% for those with nodal disease, and 14% with metastases to a distant site.

[a]Friedrich Sigmund Merkel (1845–1919) was a German anatomist and histopathologist who first described the Tastzellen (touch cells) in the skin in 1875. In 1878 the term Merkel cell was coined by the anatomist Robert Bonnet (1851–1921). Merkel cell carcinoma was first described in 1972 by Cyril Toker. He reported five cases of 'trabecular carcinoma of the skin'.

6. Overview of FDA-approved drugs for non-melanoma skin cancers

6.1. Cutaneous squamous cell carcinoma

Cemiplimab-rwlc/Libtayo

Pembrolizumab/Keytruda

6.2. Basal cell carcinoma

Aldara (Imiquimod)

Cemiplimab-rwlc

Efudex (Fluorouracil--Topical)

Erivedge (Vismodegib)

5-FU (Fluorouracil--Topical)

Fluorouracil--Topical

Imiquimod

Libtayo/Cemiplimab-rwlc)

Odomzo (Sonidegib)

Sonidegib

Vismodegib

6.3. Merkelcell carcinoma

Avelumab

Bavencio (Avelumab)

Keytruda (Pembrolizumab)

Pembrolizumab

7. Introduction to FDA-approved targeted biologic agents and specifically designed therapeutic agents for non-melanoma skin cancers

7.1. Important notes

In this section it is important to state clearly that all the information from the FDA's approved label for each biologic (which is the public domain) is taken verbatim from the label. However, I have made some minor changes to the format of each label:

i. I have brought the "DESCRIPTION" and "MECHANISM OF ACTION" sections forward to be placed immediately after the biologic's name, since how the drug works and what it is composed of, is key to understanding it.

ii. I have not generally included data from clinical trials, recommended dosage, nor recommended administration schedules, nor information on non-clinical toxicity. This book is not a clinical manual but rather aims to give an overview of the astonishing development of targeted biological agents and specifically designed therapeutic agents approved by the FDA for treatment of non-melanoma skin cancers

iii. I have put a few other salient facts in bold type to emphasize them.

iv. I have also added some material in this section that is not in the FDA approval label to illustrate certain points and to break up the many pages of words. Please note that in these cases, I have put all such added text in italics.

v. The FDA approval labels do not generally contain illustrations. All figures or images added to this section are not from the FDA label and the legends to these figures are also in italics. They are, however, are attributed in the normal way as requested by their creator.

As of December 2021, the following biological targeted agents were FDA-approved for the treatment of non-melanoma skin cancers.

8. FDA-APPROVED TARGETED BIOLOGIC THERAPEUTIC AGENTS AND SPECIFICALLY DESIGNED THERAPEUTIC AGENTS FOR NON-MELANOMA SKIN CANCERS

8.1. Cutaneous squamous cell carcinoma

Cemiplimab-rwlc/Libtayo

Pembolizumab/Keytruda

8.2. Cemiplimab-rwlc

LIBTAYO® (cemiplimab-rwlc) injection, for intravenous use

LIBTAYO is a programmed death receptor-1 (PD-1) blocking antibody indicated: Cutaneous Squamous Cell Carcinoma (CSCC)

• for the treatment of patients with metastatic cutaneous squamous cell carcinoma (mCSCC) or locally advanced CSCC (laCSCC) who are not candidates for curative surgery or curative radiation.

Basal cell carcinoma (BCC)

• for the treatment of patients with locally advanced BCC (laBCC) previously treated with a hedgehog pathway inhibitor (such as vismodegib and sonidegib), or for whom a hedgehog pathway inhibitor is not appropriate.

• for the treatment of patients with metastatic BCC (mBCC) previously treated with a hedgehog pathway inhibitor or for whom a hedgehog pathway inhibitor is not appropriate.

The mBCC indication is approved under accelerated approval based on tumor response rate and durability of response. Continued approval for mBCC may be contingent upon verification and description of clinical benefit.

(This drug is also FDA-approved for Non-Small Cell Lung Cancer (NSCLC) but this book deals only with the its use in cutaneous squamous cell carcinoma (cSCC) and basal cell carcinomaof the skin (BCC).

DESCRIPTION

Cemiplimab-rwlc is a human programmed death receptor-1 (PD-1) blocking antibody. Cemiplimab-rwlc is a recombinant human IgG4 monoclonal antibody that binds to PD-1 and blocks its interaction with PD-L1 and PD-L2. Cemiplimab-rwlc is produced by recombinant DNA technology in Chinese hamster ovary (CHO) cell suspension culture. Cemiplimab-rwlc has an approximate molecular weight of 146 kDa. LIBTAYO (cemiplimab-rwlc) injection for intravenous use is a sterile, preservative-free, clear to slightly opalescent, colorless to pale yellow solution with a pH of 6. The solution may contain trace amounts of translucent to white particles. Each vial contains 350 mg of cemiplimab-rwlc. Each mL contains cemiplimab-rwlc 50 mg, L-histidine (0.74 mg), L-histidine monohydrochloride monohydrate (1.1 mg), sucrose (50 mg), L-proline (15 mg), Polysorbate 80 (2 mg), and Water for Injection, USP.

MECHANISM OF ACTION

Binding of the PD-1 ligands PD-L1 and PD-L2, to the PD-1 receptor found on T cells, inhibits T-cell proliferation and cytokine production. Upregulation of PD-1 ligands occurs in some tumors and signaling through this pathway can contribute to inhibition of active T-cell immune surveillance of tumors. Cemiplimab-rwlc is a recombinant human immunoglobulin G4 (IgG4) monoclonal antibody that binds to PD-1 and blocks its interaction with PD-L1 and PD-L2, releasing PD-1 pathway-mediated inhibition of the immune response, including the anti-tumor immune response. In syngeneic mouse tumor models, blocking PD-1 activity resulted in decreased tumor growth.

CONTRAINDICATIONS: none.

WARNINGS AND PRECAUTIONS

Severe and fatal immune-mediated adverse reactions

LIBTAYO is a monoclonal antibody that belongs to a class of drugs that bind to either the programmed death receptor-1 (PD-1) or PD-ligand 1 (PD-L1), blocking the PD-1/PD-L1 pathway, thereby removing inhibition of the immune response, potentially breaking peripheral tolerance and inducing immune-mediated adverse reactions. Important immune-mediated adverse reactions listed under Warnings and Precautions may not include all possible severe and fatal immune-mediated reactions.

Immune-mediated adverse reactions, which may be severe or fatal, can occur in any organ system or tissue. Immune-mediated adverse reactions can occur at any time after starting PD-1/PD-L1 blocking antibody. While immune-mediated adverse reactions usually manifest during treatment with PD-1/PD-L1 blocking antibodies, immune-mediated adverse reactions can also manifest after discontinuation of PD-1/PD-L1 blocking antibodies.

Immune-mediated adverse reactions affecting more than one body system can occur simultaneously. Early identification and management of immune-mediated adverse reactions are essential to ensure safe use of PD-1/PD-L1 blocking antibodies. Monitor closely for symptoms and signs that may be clinical manifestations of underlying immune-mediated adverse reactions. Evaluate liver enzymes, creatinine, and thyroid function at baseline and periodically during treatment. In cases of suspected immune-mediated adverse reactions, initiate appropriate workup to exclude alternative etiologies, including infection. Institute medical management promptly, including specialty consultation as appropriate. Withhold or permanently discontinue LIBTAYO depending on severity. In general, if LIBTAYO requires interruption or discontinuation, administer systemic corticosteroid therapy (1 to 2 mg/kg/day prednisone or equivalent) until improvement to Grade 1 or less. Upon improvement to Grade 1 or less, initiate corticosteroid taper and continue to taper over at least 1 month. Consider administration of other systemic immunosuppressants in patients whose immune-mediated adverse reactions are not controlled with corticosteroids. Toxicity management guidelines for adverse reactions that do not necessarily require systemic steroids (e.g., endocrinopathies and dermatologic reactions) are discussed below.

Immune-mediated pneumonitis

LIBTAYO can cause immune-mediated pneumonitis. The definition of immune-mediated pneumonitis included the required use of systemic corticosteroids or other immunosuppressants and the absence of a clear alternate etiology. In patients treated with other PD-1/PD-L1 blocking antibodies the incidence of pneumonitis is higher in patients who have received **prior thoracic radiation**.

Immune-mediated pneumonitis occurred in 3.2% (26/810) of patients receiving LIBTAYO, including Grade 4 (0.5%), Grade 3 (0.5%), and Grade 2 (2.1%) adverse reactions. Pneumonitis led to permanent discontinuation of LIBTAYO in 1.4% of patients and withholding of LIBTAYO in 2.1% of the patients. Systemic corticosteroids were required in all patients with pneumonitis. Pneumonitis resolved in 58% of the 26 patients. Of the 17 patients in whom LIBTAYO was withheld for pneumonitis, 9 reinitiated LIBTAYO after symptom improvement; of these, 3/9 (33%) had recurrence of pneumonitis.

(Interstitial lung disease (ILD), or diffuse parenchymal lung disease (DPLD), is a group of lung diseases affecting the interstitium (the tissue and space around the alveoli (air sacs of the lungs) (see Figure 75). It concerns alveolar epithelium, pulmonary capillary endothelium, basement membrane, and perivascular and perilymphatic tissues. It may occur when an injury to the lungs triggers an abnormal healing response. Ordinarily, the body generates just the right

amount of tissue to repair damage, but in interstitial lung disease, the repair process goes awry and the tissue around the air sacs (alveoli) becomes scarred and thickened. This makes it more difficult for oxygen to pass into the bloodstream. The average rate of survival for someone with this disease is between three and five years. The term ILD is used to distinguish these diseases from obstructive airways diseases.

Figure 30. An alveolus (plural: alveoli, from Latin alveus, "little cavity"), is an anatomical structure that has the form of a hollow cavity. Mainly found in the lung, the pulmonary alveoli are spherical outcroppings of the respiratory bronchioles and are the primary sites of gas exchange with the blood.

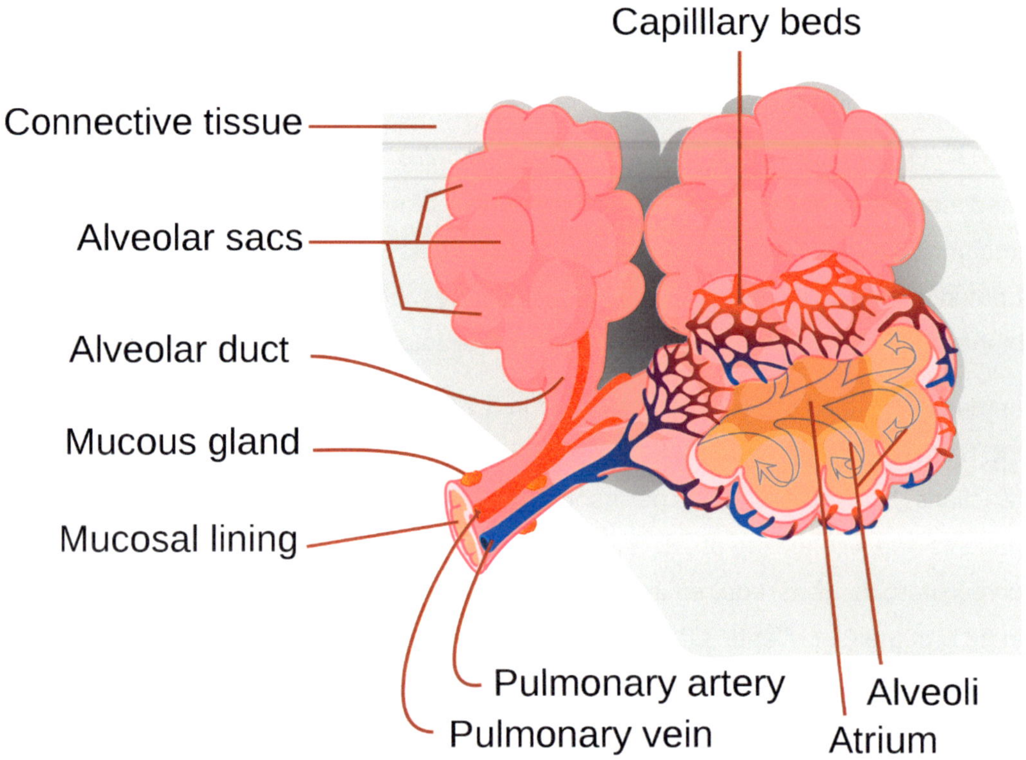

(By LadyofHats - self-made (extracted from Image:Respiratory system complete.svg) (duplicate of Image:Respiratory system complete en.svg), Public Domain, https://commons.wikimedia.org/w/index.php?curid=3222341. https://en.wikipedia.org/wiki/Interstitial_lung_disease#/media/File:Alveolus_diagram.svg. This work has been released into the public domain by its author, LadyofHats.

Figure 31 shows a photomicrograph of usual interstitial pneumonia (UIP). UIP is the most common pattern of idiopathic interstitial pneumonia (a type of interstitial lung disease) and usually represents as idiopathic pulmonary fibrosis. H&E stain. Autopsy specimen. Hyaline membranes are present.

Figure 31

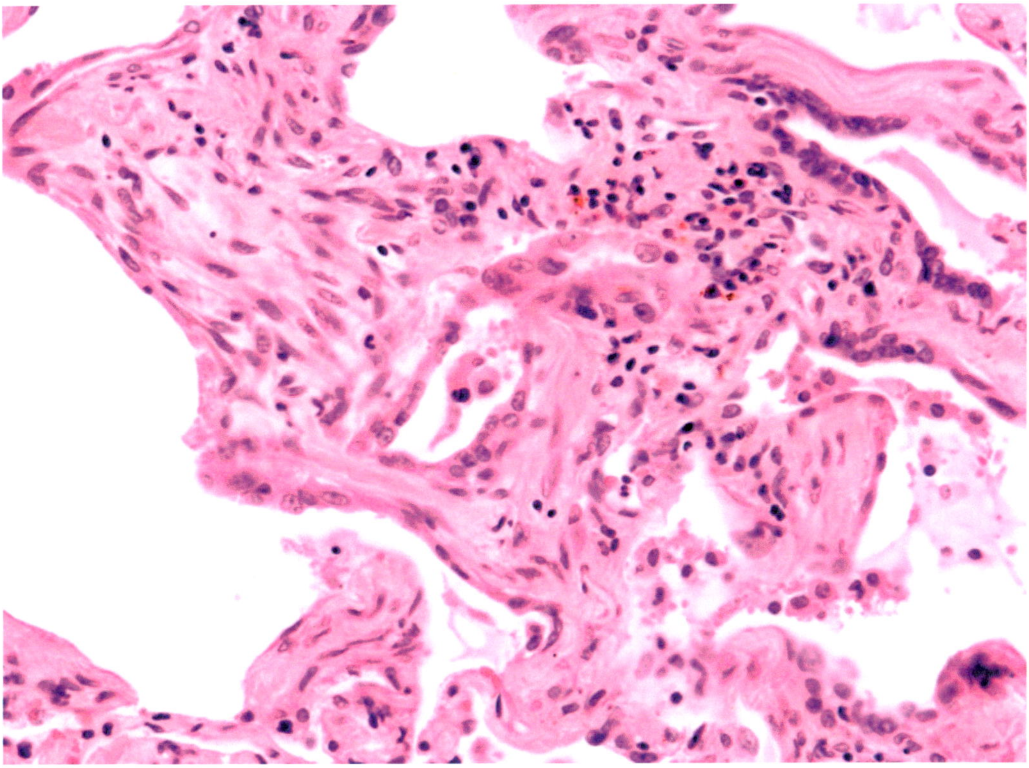

Figure 32 shows a chest x-ray of a patient with with Pneumocystis jiroveci pneumonia, showing reticular interstitial markings in all lung fields.

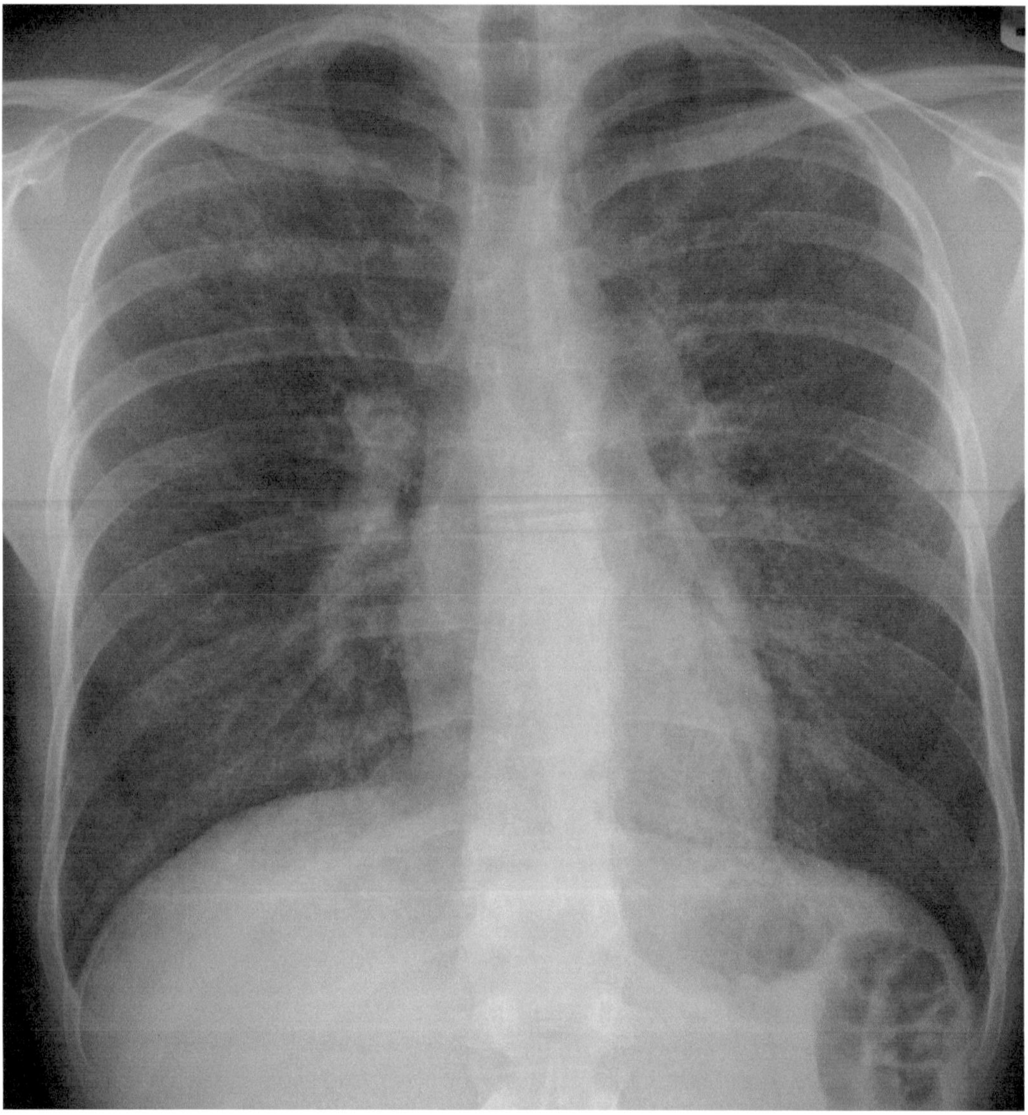

This image was released into public domain on permission of patient. -- Samir धर्म 06:38, 14 January 2007 (UTC) https://commons.wikimedia.org/w/index.php?curid=85067168. https://en.wikipedia.org/wiki/Interstitial_lung_disease#/media/File:PCP_CAP_CXR.JPG. No changes were made to this figure).

Immune-mediated colitis

LIBTAYO can cause immune-mediated colitis. The definition of immune-mediated colitis included the required use of systemic corticosteroids or other immunosuppressants and the absence of a clear alternate etiology. The primary component of the immune-mediated colitis is diarrhea. Cytomegalovirus (CMV) infection/reactivation has been reported in patients with corticosteroid-refractory immune-mediated colitis treated with PD-1/PD-L1 blocking antibodies. In cases of corticosteroid-refractory colitis, consider repeating infectious workup to exclude alternative etiologies. Immune-mediated colitis occurred in 2.2% (18/810) of patients receiving LIBTAYO, including Grade 3 (0.9%) and Grade 2 (1.1%) adverse reactions.

(Figure 33 shows the endoscopic appearance of ulcerative colitis – another cause of autoimmune colitis. Endoscopic image of ulcerative colitis affecting the left side of the colon. The image shows confluent superficial ulceration and loss of mucosal architecture.

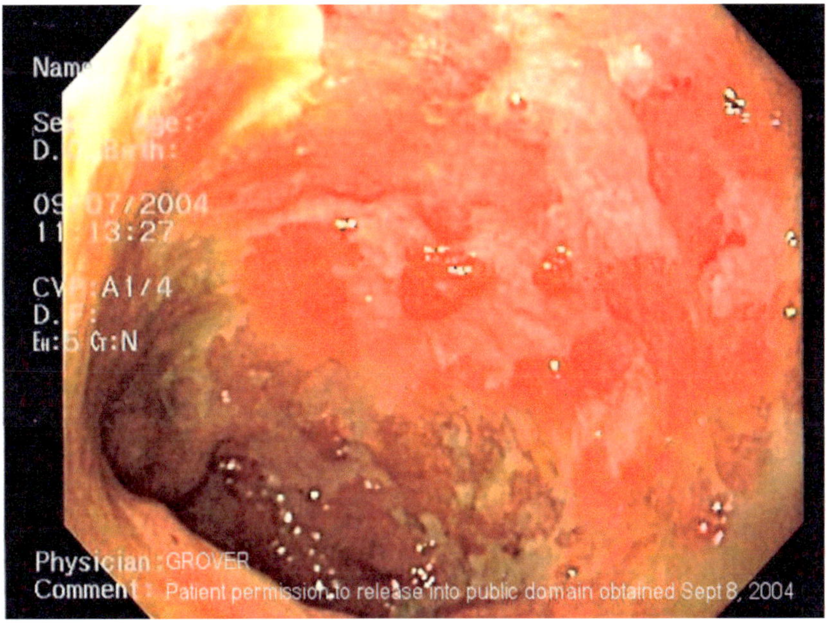

This image is by Samir at English Wikipedia, CC BY-SA 3.0, https://commons.wikimedia.org/w/index.php?curid=1002150. https://en.wikipedia.org/wiki/Ulcerative_colitis#/media/File:Ulcerative_colitis.jpg. This

file is licensed under the Creative Commons Attribution-Share Alike 3.0 Unported license. Attribution: Samir at English Wikipedia).

Colitis led to permanent discontinuation of LIBTAYO in 0.4% of patients and withholding of LIBTAYO in 1.5% of patients. Systemic corticosteroids were required in all patients with colitis. Colitis resolved in 39% of the 18 patients. Of the 12 patients in whom LIBTAYO was withheld for colitis, 4 reinitiated LIBTAYO after symptom improvement; of these, 3/4 (75%) had recurrence of colitis.

Immune-mediated hepatitis

LIBTAYO can cause immune-mediated hepatitis. The definition of immune-mediated hepatitis included the required use of systemic corticosteroids or other immunosuppressants and the absence of a clear alternate etiology. Immune-mediated hepatitis occurred in 2% (16/810) of patients receiving LIBTAYO, including fatal (0.1%), Grade 4 (0.1%), Grade 3 (1.4%), and Grade 2 (0.2%) adverse reactions. Hepatitis led to permanent discontinuation of LIBTAYO in 1.2% of patients and withholding of LIBTAYO in 0.5% of patients. Systemic corticosteroids were required in all patients with hepatitis. Nineteen percent (19%) of these patients (3/16) required additional immunosuppression with mycophenolate. Hepatitis resolved in 50% of the 16 patients. Of the 5 patients in whom LIBTAYO was withheld for hepatitis, 3 patients reinitiated LIBTAYO after symptom improvement; of these, none had recurrence of hepatitis.

(Figure 34 shows the structure of mycophenolic acid (mycophenolate).

Figure 34

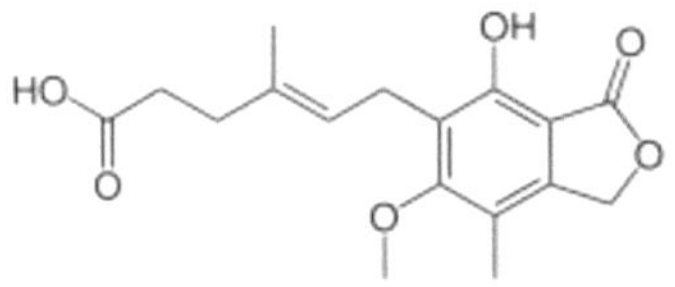

By: The original uploader was Meodipt at English Wikipedia. - Originally from en.wikipedia; description page is/was here. Public Domain, https://commons.wikimedia.org/w/index.php?curid=8401309. https://en.wikipedia.org/wiki/Mycophenolic_acid#/media/File:Mycophenolicacid.svg. No changes have been made to this image.)

Immune-mediated endocrinopathies

(As noted above, *Immunotherapy with checkpoint inhibitors has transformed the treatment of cancer, but frequently results in immune-mediated adverse events affecting multiple organs, amongst which endocrine adverse events are frequent. The patterns of endocrine adverse events differ between inhibitors of the CTLA-4 and PD-1/PD-L1 pathways, but most frequently involve the thyroid and pituitary glands with insulin-deficient diabetes also emerging as an important adverse event. These frequently result in long-lasting hormone deficiency requiring replacement.*

One study from Taiwan described immune-mediated hypophysitis in seven patients who had received immune checkpoint inhibitors for various types of advanced cancer and had received different regimens of immune checkpoint inhibitors. The time of onset after initiation of immunotherapy ranged from 5 to 36 weeks. All seven subjects were diagnosed of central adrenal insufficiency, while four of them had primary hypothyroidism. There was no typical finding of infiltrative hypophysitis on pituitary MRI. There was no documented hormone recovery after diagnosis of hypophysitis, and the tumor responses to immunotherapy were variable in these seven patients. Thus it appeared that immune-mediated hypophysitis is often irreversible. Fortunately, it also appeared to be managed adequately with hormone replacement).

Adrenal insufficiency

LIBTAYO can cause primary or secondary adrenal insufficiency. For Grade 2 or higher adrenal insufficiency, initiate symptomatic treatment, including hormone replacement as clinically indicated. Withhold LIBTAYO depending on severity. Adrenal insufficiency occurred in 0.4% (3/810) of patients receiving LIBTAYO, including Grade 3 (0.4%) adverse reactions. Adrenal insufficiency led to permanent discontinuation of LIBTAYO in 1 (0.1%) patient. Systemic corticosteroids were required in all patients with adrenal insufficiency; of these 67% (2/3) remained on systemic corticosteroids. Adrenal insufficiency had not resolved in any patient at the time of data cut-off.

Hypophysitis

LIBTAYO can cause immune-mediated hypophysitis. Hypophysitis can present with acute symptoms associated with mass effect such as headache, photophobia, or visual field defects. Hypophysitis can cause hypopituitarism. Initiate hormone replacement as clinically indicated. Withhold or permanently discontinue LIBTAYO depending on severity. Hypophysitis occurred in 0.4% (3/810) of patients receiving LIBTAYO, including Grade 3 (0.2%) and Grade 2 (0.1%) adverse reactions. Hypophysitis led to permanent discontinuation of LIBTAYO in 1 (0.1%) patient and withholding of LIBTAYO in 1 (0.1%) patient. Systemic corticosteroids were required in 67% (2/3) patients with hypophysitis. Hypophysitis had not resolved in any patient at the time of data cut-off.

(Figure 35. The anatomy of the pituitary gland.

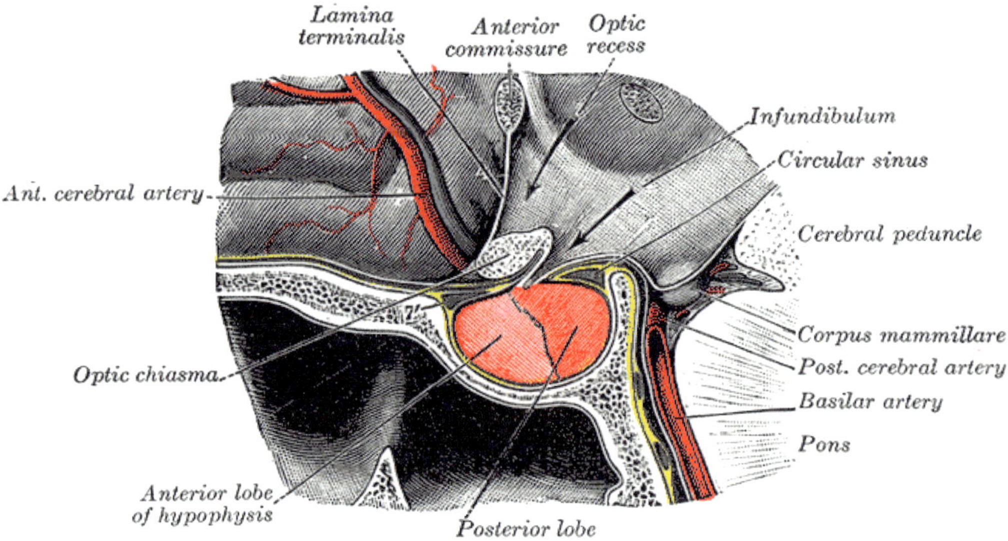

This image is by Henry Vandyke Carter - Henry Gray (1918) Anatomy of the Human Body (See "Book" section below)Bartleby.com: Gray's Anatomy, Plate 1180, Public Domain, https://commons.wikimedia.org/w/index.php?curid=567162. https://en.wikipedia.org/wiki/Hypophysitis#/media/File:Gray1180.png. This work is in the public domain in its country of origin and other countries and areas where the copyright term is the author's life plus 100 years or fewer. No changes were made to this image).

Thyroid disorders

LIBTAYO can cause immune-mediated thyroid disorders. Thyroiditis can present with or without endocrinopathy. Hypothyroidism can follow hyperthyroidism. Initiate hormone replacement or medical management of hyperthyroidism as clinically indicated. Withhold or permanently discontinue LIBTAYO depending on severity.

Thyroiditis

Thyroiditis occurred in 0.6% (5/810) of patients receiving LIBTAYO, including Grade 2 (0.2%) adverse reactions. No patient discontinued LIBTAYO due to thyroiditis. Thyroiditis led to withholding of LIBTAYO in 1 patient. Systemic corticosteroids were not required in any patient with thyroiditis. Thyroiditis had not resolved in any patient at the time of data cut-off. Blood thyroid stimulating hormone increase and blood thyroid stimulating hormone decrease have also been reported.

Hyperthyroidism

Hyperthyroidism occurred in 3.2% (26/810) of patients receiving LIBTAYO, including Grade 2 (0.9%) adverse reactions. No patient discontinued treatment due to hyperthyroidism. Hyperthyroidism led to withholding of LIBTAYO in 0.5% of patients. Systemic corticosteroids were required in 3.8% (1/26) of patients with hyperthyroidism. Hyperthyroidism resolved in 50% of the 26 patients. Of the 4 patients in whom LIBTAYO was withheld for hyperthyroidism, 2 patients reinitiated LIBTAYO after symptom improvement; of these, none had recurrence of hyperthyroidism.

Hypothyroidism

Hypothyroidism occurred in 7% (60/810) of patients receiving LIBTAYO, including Grade 2 (6%) adverse reactions. Hypothyroidism led to permanent discontinuation of LIBTAYO in 1 (0.1%) patient. Hypothyroidism led to withholding of LIBTAYO in 1.1% of patients. Systemic corticosteroids were not required in any patient with hypothyroidism. Hypothyroidism resolved in 8.3% of the 60 patients. The majority of patients with hypothyroidism required long-term thyroid hormone replacement. Of the 9 patients in whom LIBTAYO was withheld for hypothyroidism, 1 reinitiated LIBTAYO after symptom improvement; 1 required ongoing hormone replacement therapy.

Type 1 Diabetes mellitus

This can present with diabetic ketoacidosis. Monitor patients for hyperglycemia or other signs and symptoms of diabetes. Initiate treatment with insulin as clinically indicated. Withhold LIBTAYO depending on severity. Type 1 diabetes mellitus occurred in 0.1% (1/810) of patients, including Grade 4 (0.1%) adverse reactions. No patient discontinued treatment due to Type 1 diabetes mellitus. Type 1 diabetes mellitus led to withholding of LIBTAYO in 0.1% of patients.

Figure 36. Signs and symptoms of diabetes mellitus.

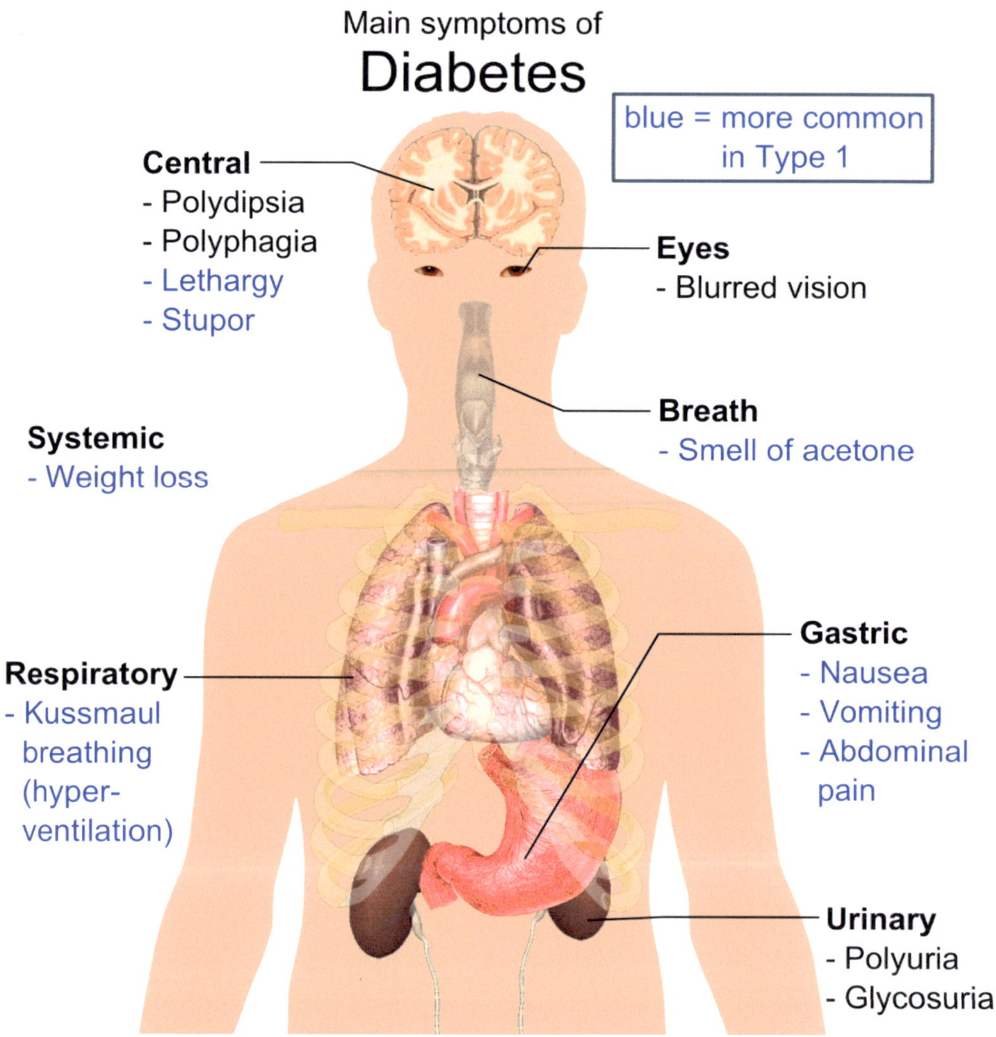

This image is by Mikael Häggström. When using this image in external works, it may be cited as: Häggström, Mikael (2014). " Medical gallery of Mikael Häggström 2014". WikiJournal of Medicine 1 (2). DOI:10.15347/wjm/2014.008. ISSN 2002-4436. Public Domain.orBy Mikael Häggström, used with permission. - See above. All used images are in public domain. Public Domain, https://commons.wikimedia.org/w/index.php?curid=6055517. https://en.wikipedia.org/wiki/Type_1_diabetes#/media/File:Main_symptoms_of_diabetes.png. Mikael Häggstrom, the copyright holder of this work, has released this work into the public domain. No changes have been made to the image).

Immune-mediated nephritis with renal dysfunction

LIBTAYO can cause immune-mediated nephritis. The definition of immune-mediated nephritis included the required use of systemic corticosteroids or other immunosuppressants and the absence of a clear alternate etiology. Immune-mediated nephritis occurred in 0.6% (5/810) patients receiving LIBTAYO, including fatal (0.1%), Grade 3 (0.1%) and Grade 2 (0.4%) adverse reactions. Nephritis led to permanent discontinuation of LIBTAYO in 0.1% of patients and withholding of LIBTAYO in 0.4% of patients. Systemic corticosteroids were required in all patients with nephritis. Nephritis resolved in 80% of the 5 patients. Of the 3 patients in whom LIBTAYO was withheld for nephritis, 2 reinitiated LIBTAYO after symptom improvement; of these, none had recurrence of nephritis.

Immune-mediated dermatologic adverse reactions

LIBTAYO can cause immune-mediated rash or dermatitis. The definition of immune-mediated dermatologic adverse reaction included the required use of systemic corticosteroids or other immunosuppressants and the absence of a clear alternate etiology.

Exfoliative dermatitis, including Stevens-Johnson Syndrome (SJS) *(Figures 37-40)*, toxic epidermal necrolysis (TEN) *(Figures 41-43)*, and DRESS (Drug Rash with Eosinophilia and Systemic Symptoms), has occurred with PD-1/PD-L1 blocking antibodies.

(Figure 37. Man with characteristic skin lesions of Stevens–Johnson syndrome.

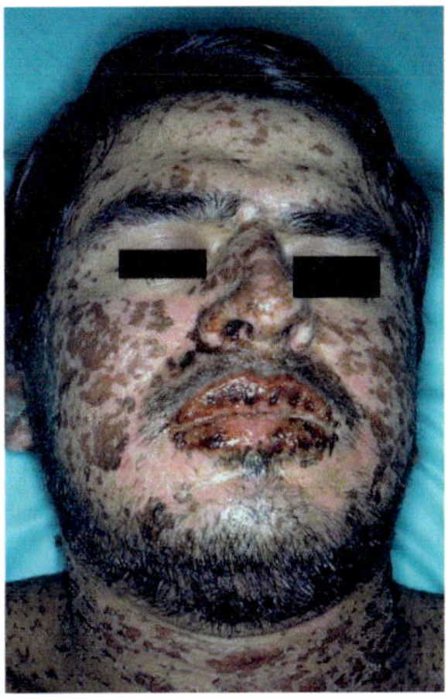

This image is by Dr. Thomas Habif - http://www.dermnet.com/Stevens-Johnson-Syndrome/picture/14975, CC BY-SA 3.0, https://commons.wikimedia.org/w/index.php?curid=9699327. https://en.wikipedia.org/wiki/Stevens%E2%80%93Johnson_syndrome#/media/File:Stevens-johnson-syndrome.jpg. This file is licensed under the Creative Commons Attribution-Share Alike 3.0 Unported license. No changes have been made to this image.

Figure 38. Mucosal desquamation in a person with Stevens–Johnson syndrome.

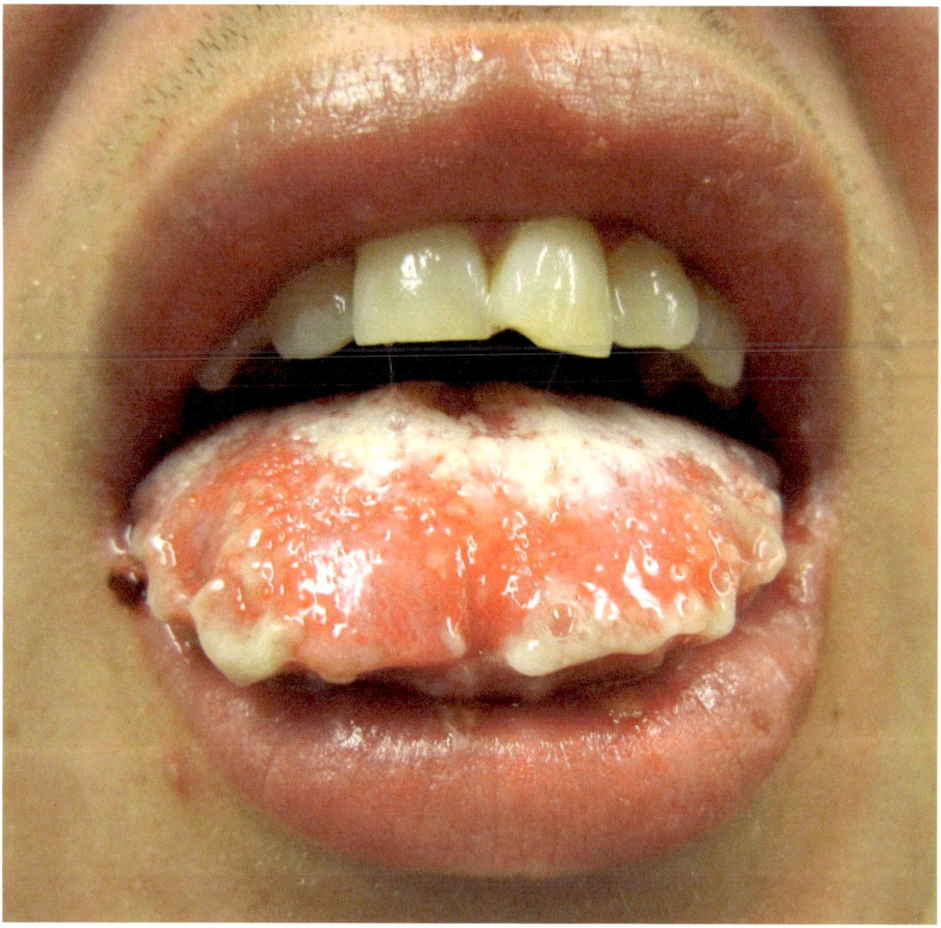

This image is by By James Heilman, MD - Own work, CC BY-SA 3.0, https://commons.wikimedia.org/w/index.php?curid=14772523. https://en.wikipedia.org/wiki/Stevens%E2%80%93Johnson_syndrome#/media/File:Mucosal_desquamation_in_a_person_with_Stevens%E2%80%93Johnson_syndrome.jpg. This file is licensed under the Creative Commons Attribution-Share Alike 3.0 Unported license. No changes have been made to this image.

Figure 39. Inflammation and peeling of the lips—with sores presenting on the tongue and the mucous membranes in Stevens-Johnson syndrome.

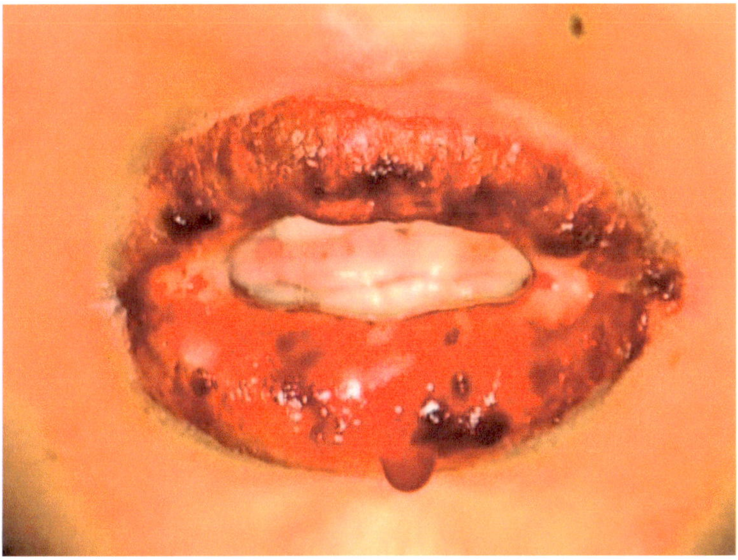

Figure 40. Conjunctivitis in Stevens-Johnson syndrome.

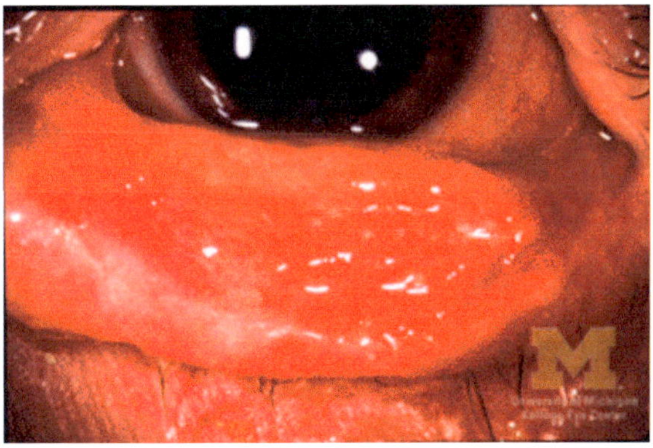

Johnson_Syndrome_Conjunctivitis.jpg. This file is licensed under the Creative Commons Attribution 3.0 Unported license. No changes have been made to this image.

Figure 41. The emerging blisters on day 4 of an instance of toxic epidermal necrolysis.

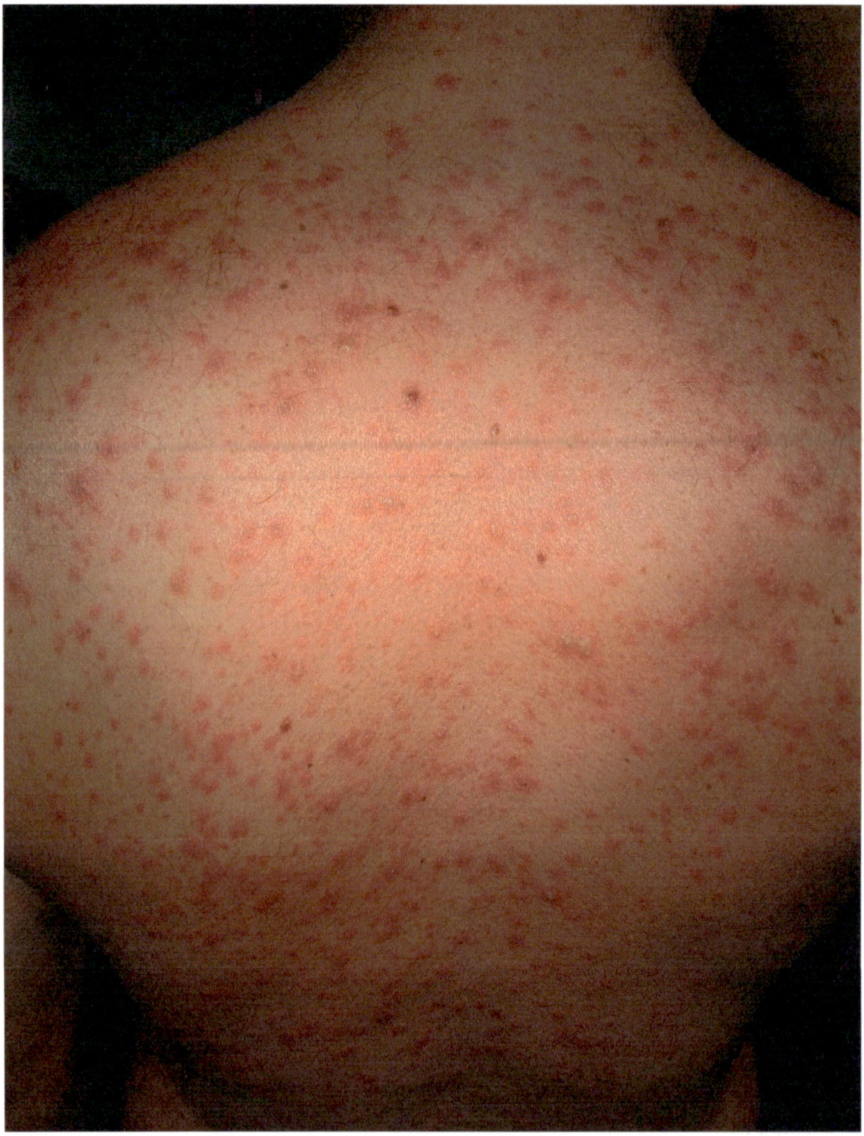

This image is by Jay2Base - Own work, CC BY-SA 4.0, https://commons.wikimedia.org/w/index.php?curid=67491052. https://en.wikipedia.org/wiki/Toxic_epidermal_necrolysis#/media/File:Early_stage_blisters_on_the_back_TENS_patient.jpg. This file is licensed under the Creative Commons Attribution-Share Alike 4.0 International license. No changes have been made to this image.

Figure 42. Toxic epidermal necrolysis.

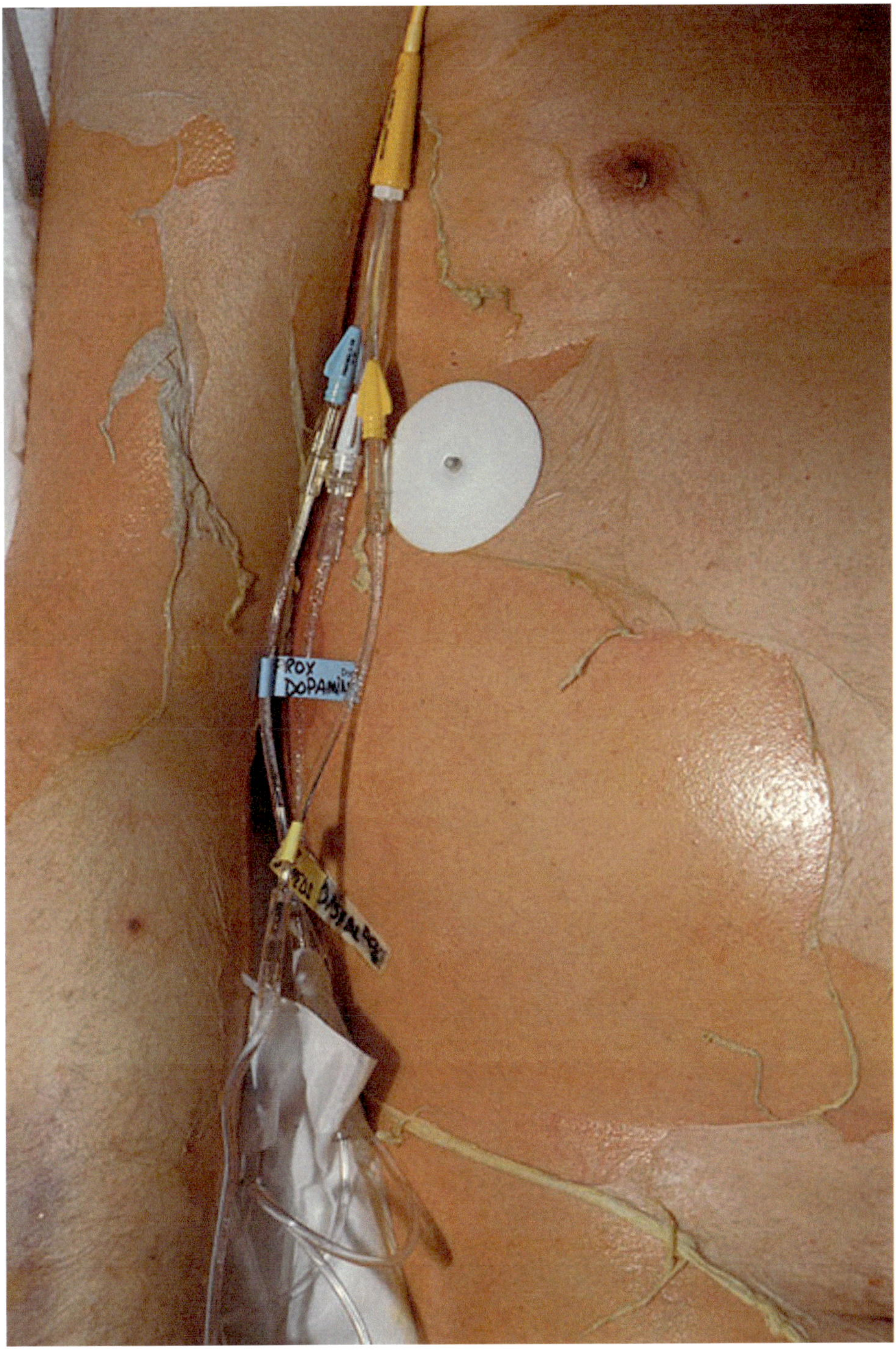

This image is by Madhero88 - http://www.dermnet.com/Toxic-Epidermal-Necrolysis/picture/14991, CC BY-SA 3.0, https://commons.wikimedia.org/w/index.php?curid=9699513. https://en.wikipedia.org/wiki/Toxic_epidermal_necrolysis#/media/File:Toxic-epidermal-necrolysis.jpg. This file is licensed under the Creative Commons Attribution-Share Alike 3.0 Unported license. No changes have been made to this image.

Figure 43. The back of a TENs patient on day 10, at the peak of the condition.

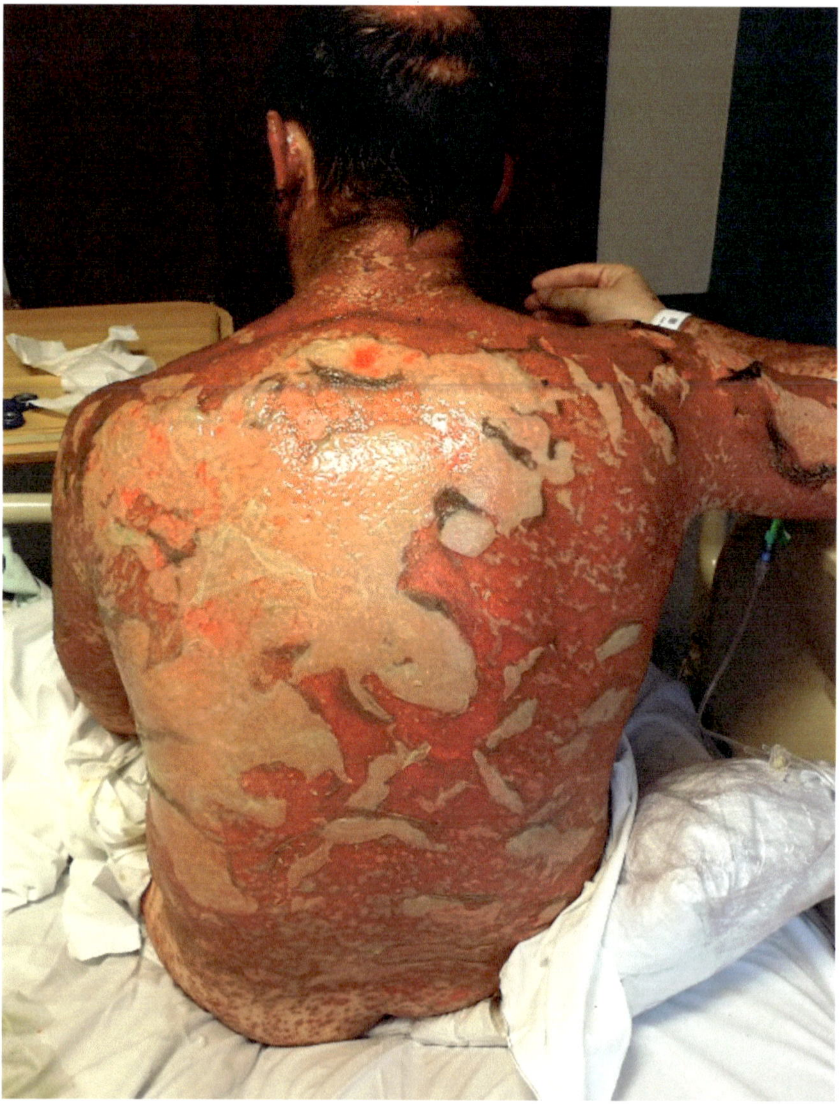

This image is by Jay2Base - Own work, CC BY-SA 4.0, https://commons.wikimedia.org/w/index.php?curid=67491133. https://en.wikipedia.org/wiki/Toxic_epidermal_necrolysis#/media/File:TENS_patient_on_day_10.jpg.

Figure 44. Histopathologic photomicrograph of confluent toxic epidermal necrolysis showing the clear separation between the epidermis and the dermis.

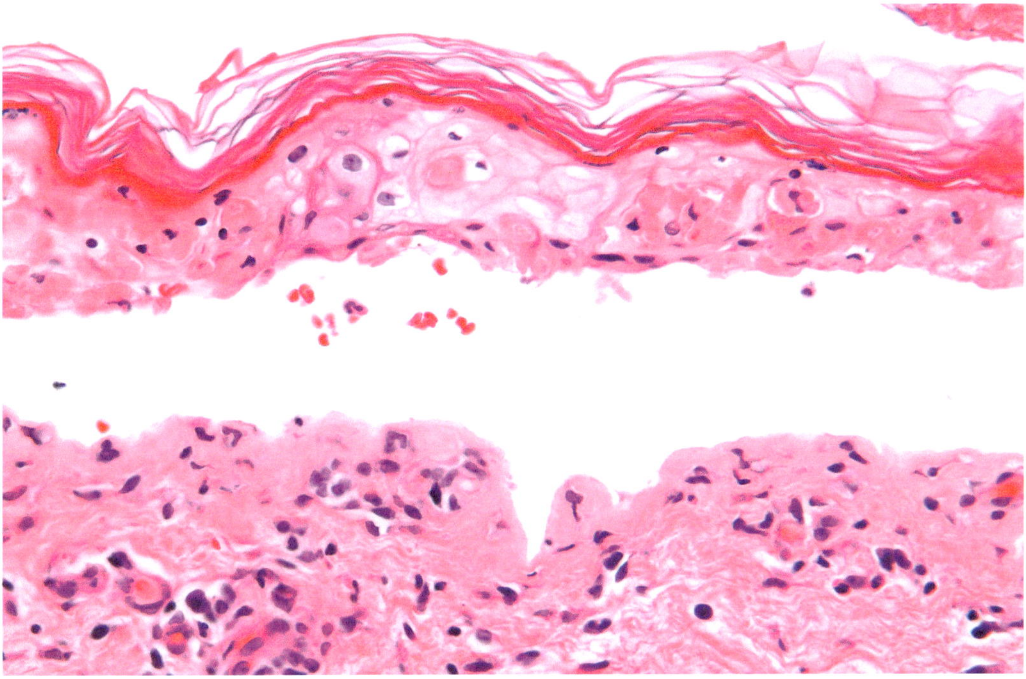

Topical emollients and/or topical corticosteroids may be adequate to treat mild to moderate non-exfoliative rashes. Withhold or permanently discontinue LIBTAYO depending on severity. Immune-mediated dermatologic adverse reactions occurred in 1.6% (13/810) of patients receiving LIBTAYO, including Grade 3 (0.9%) and Grade 2 (0.6%) adverse reactions. Dermatologic adverse reactions led to permanent discontinuation of LIBTAYO in 0.1% of patients and withholding of LIBTAYO in 1.4% of patients. Systemic corticosteroids were required in all p atients with immune-mediated dermatologic adverse reactions. Immune-mediated dermatologic adverse reactions resolved in 69% of the 13 patients. Of the 11 patients in whom LIBTAYO was withheld for dermatologic adverse reaction, 7 reinitiated LIBTAYO after symptom improvement; of these 43% (3/7) had recurrence of the dermatologic adverse reaction.

Other immune-mediated adverse reactions

The following clinically significant immune-mediated adverse reactions occurred at an incidence of < 1% in 810 patients who received LIBTAYO or were reported with the use of other PD-1/PD-L1 blocking antibodies. Severe or fatal cases have been reported for some of these adverse reactions.

Cardiac/Vascular: myocarditis, pericarditis, vasculitis

Nervous System: meningitis, encephalitis, myelitis and demyelination, myasthenic syndrome / myasthenia gravis (including exacerbation), Guillain-Barre syndrome, nerve paresis, autoimmune neuropathy

Ocular: uveitis, iritis, and other ocular inflammatory toxicities. Some cases can be associated with retinal detachment. Various grades of visual impairment to include blindness can occur. If uveitis occurs in combination with other immune-mediated adverse reactions, consider a Vogt-Koyanagi-Harada like syndrome, as this may require treatment with systemic steroids to reduce the risk of permanent vision loss.

Gastrointestinal: pancreatitis to include increases in serum amylase and lipase levels, gastritis, duodenitis, stomatitis

Musculoskeletal and connective tissue: myositis/polymyositis, rhabdomyolysis and associated sequelae including renal failure, arthritis, polymyalgia rheumatica

Endocrine: hypoparathyroidism

Other (hematologic/immune): hemolytic anemia, aplastic anemia, hemophagocytic lymphohistiocytosis, systemic inflammatory response syndrome, histiocytic necrotizing lymphadenitis (Kikuchi lymphadenitis), sarcoidosis, immune thrombocytopenic purpura, solid organ transplant rejection.

Infusion-related reactions

Severe infusion-related reactions (Grade 3) occurred in 0.1% of patients receiving LIBTAYO as a single agent. Monitor patients for signs and symptoms of infusion-related reactions. The most common symptoms of infusion-related reaction were nausea, pyrexia, rash and dyspnea. Interrupt or slow the rate of infusion or permanently discontinue LIBTAYO based on severity of reaction.

Complications of allogeneic hematopoietic stem cell transplantation (HSCT)

Fatal and other serious complications can occur in patients who receive allogeneic hematopoietic stem cell transplantation (HSCT) before or after being treated with a PD-1/PD-L1 blocking antibody. Transplant-related complications include hyperacute graft-versus-host-disease (GVHD), acute GVHD, chronic GVHD, hepatic veno-occlusive disease (VOD) after reduced intensity conditioning, and steroid-requiring febrile syndrome (without an identified infectious cause). These complications may occur despite intervening therapy between PD-1/PD-L1 blockade and allogeneic HSCT. Follow patients closely for evidence of transplant-related complications and intervene promptly. Consider the benefit versus risks of treatment with a PD-1/PD-L1 blocking antibody prior to or after an allogeneic HSCT.

Embryo-fetal toxicity

Based on its mechanism of action, LIBTAYO can cause fetal harm when administered to a pregnant woman. Animal studies have demonstrated that inhibition of the PD-1/PD-L1 pathway can lead to increased risk of immune-mediated rejection of the developing fetus resulting in fetal death. Advise women of the potential risk to a fetus. Advise females of reproductive potential to use effective contraception during treatment with LIBTAYO and for at least 4 months after the last dose.

Immunogenicity

As with all therapeutic proteins, there is a potential for immunogenicity. The detection of antibody formation is highly dependent on the sensitivity and specificity of the assay. Additionally, the observed incidence of antibody (including neutralizing antibody) positivity in an assay may be influenced by several factors including assay methodology, sample handling, timing of sample collection, concomitant medications, and underlying disease. For these reasons, comparison of the incidence of antibodies to cemiplimab-rwlc in the studies described below with the incidence of antibodies in other studies or to other products may be misleading. Anti-drug antibodies (ADA) were tested in 823 patients who received LIBTAYO. The incidence of cemiplimab-rwlc treatment-emergent ADAs was 2.2% using an electrochemiluminescent (ECL) bridging immunoassay; 0.4% were persistent ADA responses. In the patients who developed anti-cemiplimab-rwlc antibodies, there was no evidence of an altered pharmacokinetic profile of cemiplimab-rwlc.

USE IN SPECIFIC POPULATIONS

Pregnancy risk summary

Based on its mechanism of action, LIBTAYO can cause fetal harm when administered to a pregnant woman. There are no available data on the use of LIBTAYO in pregnant women. Animal studies have demonstrated that inhibition of the PD-1/PD-L1 pathway can lead to increased risk of immune-mediated rejection of the developing fetus resulting in fetal death (see Data). Human IgG4 immunoglobulins (IgG4) are known to cross the placenta; therefore, LIBTAYO has the potential to be transmitted from the mother to the developing fetus. Advise women of the potential risk to a fetus. In the U.S. general population, the estimated background risk of major birth defects and miscarriage in clinically recognized pregnancies is 2% to 4% and 15% to 20%, respectively.

Data

Animal data

Animal reproduction studies have not been conducted with LIBTAYO to evaluate its effect on reproduction and fetal development. A central function of the PD-1/PD-L1 pathway is to preserve pregnancy by maintaining maternal immune tolerance to the fetus. In murine models of pregnancy, blockade of PD-L1 signaling has been shown to disrupt tolerance to the fetus and to result in an increase in fetal loss; therefore, potential risks of administering LIBTAYO during pregnancy include increased rates of abortion or stillbirth. As reported in the literature, there were no malformations related to the blockade of PD-1/PD-L1 signaling in the offspring of these animals; however, immune-mediated disorders occurred in PD-1 and PD-L1 knockout mice. Based on its mechanism of action, fetal exposure to cemiplimab-rwlc may increase the risk of developing immune-mediated disorders or altering the normal immune response.

Lactation risk summary

There is no information regarding the presence of cemiplimab-rwlc in human milk, or its effects on the breastfed child or on milk production. Because of the potential for serious adverse reactions in breastfed children, advise women not to breastfeed during treatment and for at least 4 months after the last dose of LIBTAYO.

Females and males of reproductive potential

Pregnancy Testing

Verify pregnancy status in females of reproductive potential prior to initiating LIBTAYO.

Contraception

LIBTAYO can cause fetal harm when administered to a pregnant woman.

Females

Advise females of reproductive potential to use effective contraception during treatment with LIBTAYO and for at least 4 months after the last dose.

Pediatric use

The safety and effectiveness of LIBTAYO have not been established in pediatric patients.

Geriatric use

Of the 810 patients who received LIBTAYO in clinical studies, 32% were 65 years up to 75 years and 22% were 75 years or older. No overall differences in safety or effectiveness were observed between these patients and younger patients. Of the 219 patients with mCSCC or laCSCC who received LIBTAYO in clinical studies, 34% were 65 years up to 75 years and 41% were 75 years or older. No overall differences in safety or effectiveness were observed between these patients and younger patients. Of the 132 patients with BCC who received LIBTAYO in Study 1620, 27% were 65 years up to 75 years, and 32% were 75 years or older. No overall differences in safety or effectiveness were observed between these patients and younger patients.

Pharmacokinetics

Cemiplimab-rwlc pharmacokinetic data were collected in 1062 patients with various solid tumors in a population pharmacokinetic analysis. The pharmacokinetics of cemiplimab-rwlc were linear and dose proportional in the dose range of 1 mg/kg to 10 mg/kg LIBTAYO administered intravenously every 2 weeks. At 350 mg every 3 weeks, the mean cemiplimab-rwlc concentrations (coefficient of variation, CV%) at steady-state ranged between a minimum concentration of 61 mg/L (45%) and a maximum concentration of 171 mg/L (28%). Steady-state exposure is achieved after 4 months of treatment. In patients with CSCC, cemiplimab-rwlc steady-state exposure at 350 mg every 3 weeks was comparable to the exposure at 3 mg/kg every 2 weeks.

Distribution

The volume of distribution of cemiplimab-rwlc at steady state is 5.3 L (26%).

Elimination

Cemiplimab-rwlc clearance (CV%) after the first dose is 0.29 L/day (33%) and decreases over time by 29%, resulting in a steady-state clearance (CLss) (CV%) of 0.20 L/day (40%). The elimination half-life (CV%) at steady state is 20.3 days (29%).

Specific populations

The following factors have no clinically important effect on the exposure of cemiplimab-rwlc: age (27 to 96 years), sex, body weight (31 to 172 kg), cancer type, albumin level (20 to 93 g/L), renal function (creatinine clearance determined by Cockcroft-Gault 21 mL/min or greater) and hepatic function (total bilirubin greater than 1.0 times up to 3.0 times the ULN). Race [White (N=931), Black (N=47), Asian (N=21)] appears to have no clinically important effect on the exposure of cemiplimab-rwlc. LIBTAYO has not been studied in patients with severe hepatic impairment.

8.3. Keytruda/pembrolizumab

KEYTRUDA® (pembrolizumab) for injection, for intravenous use.

Pembrolizumab is a programmed death receptor-1 (PD 1)-blocking antibody. Pembrolizumab is a humanized monoclonal IgG4 kappa antibody with an approximate molecular weight of 149 kDa. Pembrolizumab is produced in recombinant Chinese hamster ovary (CHO) cells.

Keytruda is FDA-approved for many diseases including cutaneous Squamous Cell Carcinoma (cSCC)

- for the treatment of patients with recurrent or metastatic cutaneous squamous cell carcinoma that is not curable by surgery or radiation.

Mechanism of action

Binding of the PD-1 ligands, PD-L1 and PD-L2, to the PD-1 receptor found on T cells, inhibits T cell proliferation and cytokine production. Upregulation of PD-1 ligands occurs in some tumors and signaling through this pathway can contribute to inhibition of active T-cell immune surveillance of tumors. Pembrolizumab is a monoclonal antibody that binds to the PD-1 receptor and blocks its interaction with PD-L1 and PD-L2, releasing PD-1 pathway-mediated inhibition of the immune response, including the anti-tumor immune response. In syngeneic mouse tumor models, blocking PD-1 activity resulted in decreased tumor growth.

(A space-filling model of pembrolizumab is shown in Figure 45. False-colored to more easily distinguish heavy and light chains. Style made to resemble the Protein Data Bank's "Molecule of the Month" series, illustrated by Dr. David S. Goodsell of the Scripps Research Institute. Created using QuteMol (http://qutemol.sourceforge.net). Optimized with OptiPNG.

This image is in the public domain because its creator has placed it there. By Fvasconcellos (talk · contribs) - From PDB entry 5DK3. More information:Scapin G, Yang X, Prosise WW, et al. Structure of full-length human anti-PD1 therapeutic IgG4 antibody pembrolizumab. Nat Struct Mol Biol 2015;22(12):953-8. doi:10.1038/nsmb.3129, Public Domain,https://commons.wikimedia.org/w/index.php?curid=61341750. https://en.wikipedia.org/wiki/Pembrolizumab#/media/File:Pembrolizumab_5DK3.png)

Figure 45

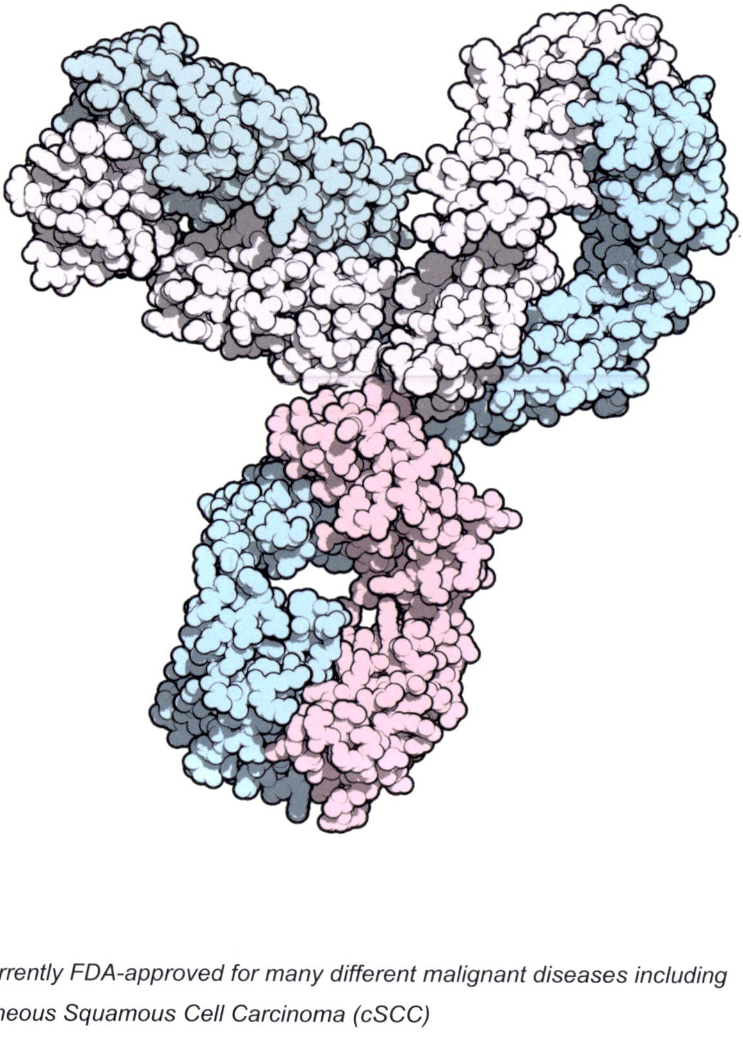

Keytruda is currently FDA-approved for many different malignant diseases including including cutaneous Squamous Cell Carcinoma (cSCC)

CONTRAINDICATIONS: none.

WARNINGS AND PRECAUTIONS

• Immune-mediated pneumonitis: **withhold for moderate, and permanently discontinue for severe, life-threatening or recurrent moderate pneumonitis.**

• Immune-mediated colitis: **withhold for moderate or severe, and permanently discontinue for life-threatening colitis.**

• Immune-mediated hepatitis (KEYTRUDA) and hepatotoxicity (KEYTRUDA in combination with axitinib): monitor for changes in hepatic function. Based on severity of liver enzyme elevations, withhold or discontinue KEYTRUDA, axitinib, or KEYTRUDA and axitinib. Consider corticosteroid therapy.

• Immune-mediated endocrinopathies

o Adrenal insufficiency: **withhold for moderate and withhold or permanently discontinue for severe or life-threatening adrenal insufficiency.**

o Hypophysitis: **withhold for moderate and withhold or permanently discontinue for severe or life-threatening hypophysitis.**

o Thyroid disorders: monitor for changes in thyroid function. **Withhold or permanently discontinue for severe or lifethreatening hyperthyroidism.**

o Type 1 diabetes mellitus: monitor for hyperglycemia. Withhold KEYTRUDA in cases of severe hyperglycemia.

• Immune-mediated nephritis: monitor for changes in renal function**. Withhold for moderate, and permanently discontinue for severe or life-threatening nephritis.**

• Immune-mediated skin adverse reactions including Stevens-Johnson syndrome (SJS) and toxic epidermal necrolysis (TEN): **withhold for severe and permanently discontinue for life-threatening skin reactions.**

Other immune-mediated adverse reactions: in organ transplant recipients, consider the benefit of treatment with KEYTRUDA versus the risk of possible organ rejection.
• Infusion-related reactions: **stop infusion and permanently discontinue KEYTRUDA for severe or life-threatening infusion reactions**.

• Complications of allogeneic hematopoietic stem cell transplantation (HSCT)

o Allogeneic HSCT after treatment with KEYTRUDA: monitor for hepatic veno-occlusive disease (also known as hepatic sinusoidal obstruction syndrome), grade 3-4 acute graft-versus-host disease (GVHD) including hyperacute GVHD, steroid-requiring febrile syndrome, and other immune-mediated adverse reactions. Transplant-related mortality has occurred.

o Allogeneic HSCT prior to treatment with KEYTRUDA: in patients with a history of allogeneic HSCT, consider the benefit of treatment with KEYTRUDA versus the risk of GVHD.

• Treatment of patients with multiple myeloma with a PD-1 or PD-L1 blocking antibody in combination with a thalidomide analogue plus dexamethasone is not recommended outside of controlled clinical trials.

• Embryo-fetal toxicity: can cause fetal harm. Advise females of reproductive potential of the potential risk to a fetus and to use an effective method of contraception.

(Immune-mediated pneumonitis (IMP) is an uncommon but potentially fatal toxicity of anti–programmed death-1 (PD-1)/programmed death ligand 1 (PD-L1) therapy for cancer. In one study several CT findings including diffuse reticulation, patchy/diffuse ground glass opacification, and interlobular septal thickening with bilateral and peripheral distribution were more frequent in IMP than pneumonia by pathogen. Clinical findings overlapped).

• Immune-mediated hepatitis: monitor for changes in liver function. **Withhold or permanently discontinue based on severity of transaminase or total bilirubin elevation.**

(Immune-mediated hepatitis is defined as an elevation in the patient's liver function tests that requires corticosteroids and that has no alternate etiology. It can be the result of autoimmune hepatitis or be caused by immunotherapeutic treatments for cancer such as anti-PD-1L agents including avelumab, durvalumab and atezolizumab)

• Immune-mediated colitis**: withhold or permanently discontinue based on severity of colitis.**

(Immune-mediated colitis (IMC) is a common immune related adverse event associated with immune checkpoint inhibitors (ICIs). It typically occurs 5 -10 weeks

after the 2nd or 3rd dose of treatment with the immune checkpoint inhibitor. Endoscopically it is indistinguishable from inflammatory bowel disease with a significant overlap in histology. Optimal management of IMC requires early recognition and timely use of corticosteroids. About one third to two thirds of patients are steroid-refractory. ***Infliximab*** *is the second line therapy in these patients. Recent reports have shown that* ***vedolizumab*** *is more gut-specific and efficacious in steroid- and infliximab-refractory cases. To date there are 7 approved checkpoint inhibitors that target 3 main checkpoints, including cytotoxic T-lymphocyte associated protein 4 (CTLA-4; ipilimumab and tremelimumab), programmed cell death receptor 1 (PD-1; pembrolizumab and nivolumab), and programmed death ligand 1 (PD-L1; atezolizumab, avelumab, and durvalumab). While representing a remarkable breakthrough in the treatment of several advanced malignancies, several ICI-related adverse events that affect multiple body systems have been recognized).*

• Immune-mediated endocrinopathies

(Immunotherapy with checkpoint inhibitors has transformed the treatment of cancer, but frequently results in immune-mediated adverse events affecting multiple organs, amongst which endocrine adverse events are frequent. The patterns of endocrine adverse events differ between inhibitors of the CTLA-4 and PD-1/PD-L1 pathways, but most frequently involve the thyroid and pituitary with insulin-deficient diabetes also emerging as an important adverse event. These frequently result in long-lasting hormone deficiency requiring replacement).

o Hypophysitis: withhold based on severity of hypophysitis

(One study from Taiwan described immune-mediated hypophysitis in seven patients who had received immune checkpoint inhibitors for various types of advanced cancer and had received different regimens of immune checkpoint inhibitors. The time of onset after initiation of immunotherapy ranged from 5 to 36 weeks. All seven subjects were diagnosed of central adrenal insufficiency, while four of them had primary hypothyroidism. There was no typical finding of infiltrative hypophysitis on pituitary MRI. There was no documented hormone recovery after diagnosis of hypophysitis, and the tumor responses to immunotherapy were variable in these seven patients. Thus it appeared that immune-mediated hypophysitis is often

irreversible. Fortunately, it also appeared to be managed adequately with hormone replacement).

o Thyroid disorders: monitor for changes in thyroid function. Withhold based on severity of hyperthyroidism.

o Adrenal insufficiency: withhold based on severity of adrenal insufficiency.

o Type 1 diabetes mellitus: withhold based on severity of hyperglycemia.

- Infections: withhold for severe or life-threatening infection
- Infusion-related reactions: **interrupt, slow the rate of infusion, or permanently discontinue based on severity of infusion reactions.**
- Embryo-fetal toxicity: can cause fetal harm. Advise females of reproductive potential of the potential risk to a fetus and use of effective contraception

ADVERSE REACTIONS

- Most common adverse reactions (reported in ≥ 20% of patients) with TECENTRIQ as a single-agent were fatigue/asthenia, nausea, cough, dyspnea, and decreased appetite
- Most common adverse reactions (reported in ≥ 20% of patients) with TECENTRIQ in combination with other antineoplastic drugs in patients with NSCLC and SCLC were fatigue/asthenia, nausea, alopecia, constipation, diarrhea, and decreased appetite

USE IN SPECIFIC POPULATIONS

Lactation: advise not to breastfeed.

Pediatric use: the safety and effectiveness of TECENTRIQ have not been established in pediatric patients.

Geriatric use: of 2481 patients with urothelial carcinoma, lung cancer, and triple-negative breast cancer who 654 were treated with TECENTRIQ in clinical studies, 45% were 65 years and over and 11% were 655 75 years and over. No overall differences in safety or effectiveness were observed between 656 patients aged 65 years or older, and younger patients.

Other immune-mediated disorders: if uveitis occurs in combination with other immune-mediated adverse reactions, evaluate for Vogt-Koyanagi-Harada syndrome, which has been observed with other products in this class and may require treatment with systemic steroids to reduce the risk of permanent vision loss. The following clinically significant, immune-mediated adverse reactions occurred at an incidence of < 1% in 2616 patients who received TECENTRIQ as a single-agent and in 2421 patients who received TECENTRIQ in combination with platinum-based chemotherapy or were reported in other products in this class.

Dermatologic

Bullous dermatitis, pemphigoid, erythema multiforme, Stevens-Johnson Syndrome (SJS)/toxic epidermal necrolysis (TEN)

(Immune-mediated bullous disorders include pemphigus vulgaris, pemphigoid, dermatitis herpetiformis and linear immunoglobulin-A disease (Figures 46-49)

(Figure 46. Pemphigus vulgaris)

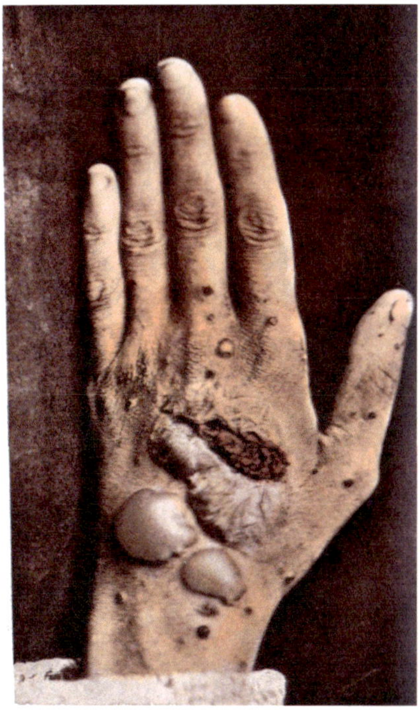

(This image, reproduced here from Wikimedia Commons, shows large blisters on the dorsum of the hand typical of pemphigus vulgaris).

(https://commons.wikimedia.org/wiki/File:Permphigus.jpg. This media file is in the public domain in the United States. This applies to U.S. works where the copyright has expired, often because its first publication occurred prior to January 1, 1925 (PD 1925). Source: Fox, George Henry (1886) Photographic illustrations of skin diseases). No changes were made to this image).

(Figure 47. Pemphigoid. The blisters are tense, about 1–4 cm in diameter, leaving eroded and crusted areas.

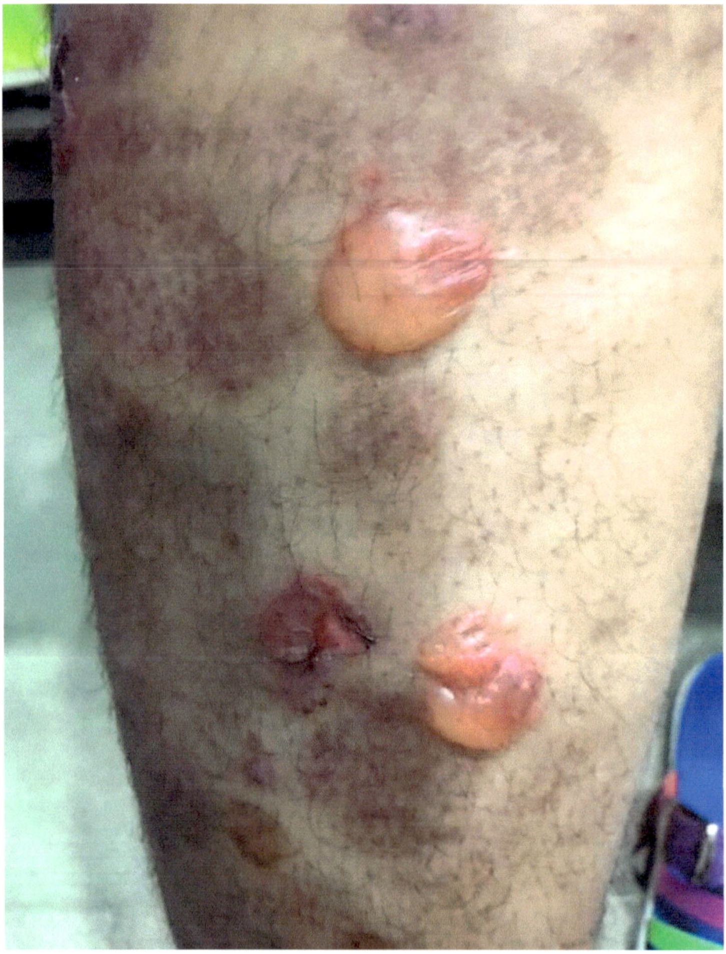

This image is by Mohammad2018 - Own work, CC BY-SA 4.0, By Mohammad2018 - Own work, CC BY-SA 4.0, https://commons.wikimedia.org/w/index.php?curid=73315087. https://en.wikipedia.org/wiki/Pemphigoid#/media/File:Bullous_pemphigoid_new_imag

e.jpg. This image is licensed under the Creative Commons Attribution-Share Alike 4.0 International license. https://creativecommons.org/licenses/by-sa/4.0/deed.en. No changes were made to this image).

(Figure 48. Dermatitis herpetiformis)

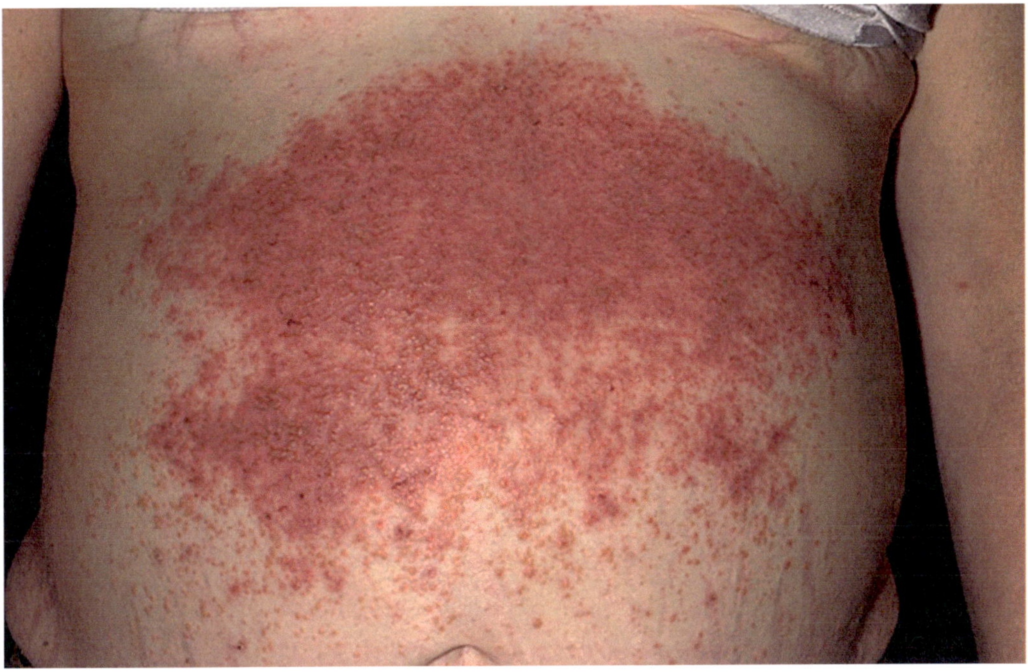

(The characteristic rash resembles herpes and is the basis of its clinical name, although the disease is not caused by, or related to, herpes except for the appearance of the blisters. By Madhero88 - http://www.dermnet.com/Dermatitis-Herpetiformis/picture/13646, CC BY-SA 3.0, https://commons.wikimedia.org/w/index.php?curid=9700760.Thomas Habif authorises the use of the 21 pictures listed here and published on the website dermnet.com under the license Creative Commons Attribution ShareAlike 3.0. https://commons.wikimedia.org/wiki/File:Dermatitis-herpetiformis.jpg. https://creativecommons.org/licenses/by-sa/3.0/. No changes were made to this image).

(Figure 49. Linear immunoglobulin A disease)

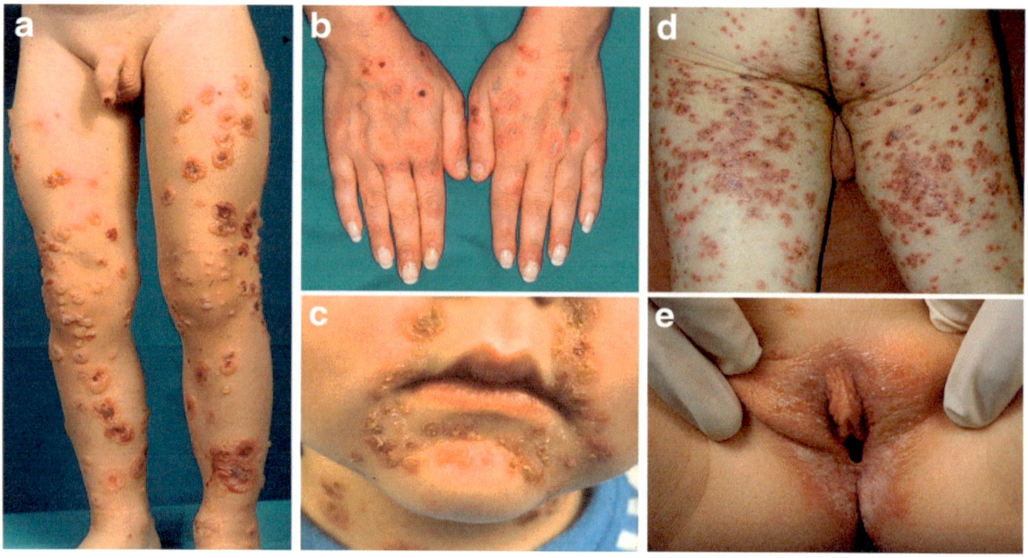

(Linear IgA bullous dermatosis:

a Widespread vesiculobullous eruption on the lower limbs with elements in a "string of pearls" arrangement;

(b) targetoid vesicular lesions on erythematous skin involving the dorsa of the hands;

(c) blisters with a "string of pearls" configuration and crusts in the perioral area;

(d) erythematous, vesicular lesions partially eroded on the posterior aspects of both thighs;

(e) vesicles involving the vulvar area in a child

By Giovanni Genovese, Luigia Venegoni, Daniele Fanoni, Simona Muratori, Emilio Berti, Angelo Valerio Marzano - (2019). "Linear IgA bullous dermatosis in adults and children: a clinical and immunopathological study of 38 patients". Orphanet Journal of Rare Diseases 14 (1). DOI:10.1186/s13023-019-1089-2. ISSN 1750-1172."This article is distributed under the terms of the Creative Commons Attribution 4.0 International License (http://creativecommons.org/licenses/by/4.0/)", CC BY 4.0, https://commons.wikimedia.org/w/index.php?curid=83709527: https://en.wikipedia.org/wiki/Linear_IgA_bullous_dermatosis#/media/File:Linear_IgA_bullous_dermatosis.jpg. No changes were made to this image)

(Figure 50. Erythema multiforme)

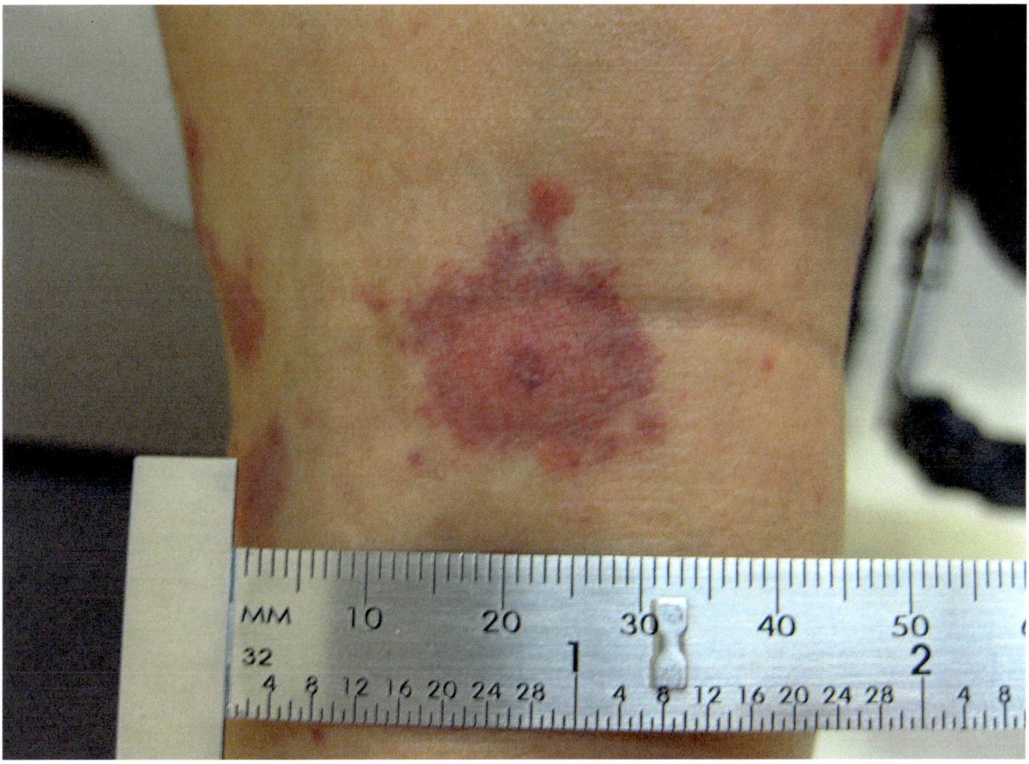

(An erythema multiforme lesion showing the classical "target lesion" appearance, with a pink-red ring around a pale center. By kilbad (talk) - I (kilbad (talk)) created this work entirely by myself., CC BY-SA 3.0, https://en.wikipedia.org/w/index.php?curid=23658508. https://en.wikipedia.org/wiki/Erythema_multiforme#/media/File:Target_lesion_1.jpg. This work is licensed under the Creative Commons Attribution-ShareAlike). 3.0 License. No changes were made to this image.

(Stevens-Johnson Syndrome [SJS] and toxic epidermal necrolysis [TEN]. This is a spectrum of disease with toxic epidermal necrolysis being the more severe form.

Gastrointestinal: pancreatitis, including increases in serum amylase or lipase levels.
General: systemic inflammatory response syndrome, histiocytic necrotizing lymphadenitis

ADVERSE REACTIONS

The most common adverse reactions (reported in ≥20% of patients) were:

• KEYTRUDA as a single agent: fatigue, musculoskeletal pain, decreased appetite, pruritus, diarrhea, nausea, rash, pyrexia, cough, dyspnea, constipation, pain, and abdominal pain.

KEYTRUDA in combination with chemotherapy: fatigue/asthenia, nausea, constipation, diarrhea, decreased appetite, rash, vomiting, cough, dyspnea, pyrexia, alopecia, peripheral neuropathy, mucosal inflammation, and stomatitis.

• KEYTRUDA in combination with axitinib: *(axitinib is a selective tyrosine kinase inhibitor (TKI) of vascular endothelial growth factor (VEGR) receptors 1, 2 and 3. These receptors are implicated in pathological angiogenesis, tumour growth and metastatic progression of cancer. It is FDA-approved for the treatment of advanced renal cell carcinoma after failure of one prior systemic therapy).*

diarrhea, fatigue/asthenia, hypertension, hepatotoxicity, hypothyroidism, decreased appetite**, palmar-plantar erythrodysesthesia**, nausea, stomatitis/mucosal inflammation, dysphonia, rash, cough, and constipation.

(Palmar-plantar erythrodysesthesia is reddening, swelling, numbness and desquamation (skin sloughing or peeling) on the palms of the hands and soles of the feet (and, occasionally, on the knees, elbows, and elsewhere). It can also occur after chemotherapy in patients with cancer , when it is known as chemotherapy-induced acral erythema or hand-foot syndrome. The skin changes are usually well demarcated (Figure 40). Acral erythema typically disappears within a few weeks after discontinuation of the offending drug).

(Figure 51. Chemotherapy-induced acral erythema/ palmar-plantar erythrodysesthesia. Picture of the palms of the hands after about 10 days of capecitabine (chemotherapy) showing signs of medium-severe chemotherapy-induced acral erythema (hand-foot syndrome). This image, reproduced here from Wikimedia Commons, is in the public domain because its creator has placed it there. By Lucid Smog (Lucid Smog (talk)) - Own work, Public Domain, https://commons.wikimedia.org/w/index.php?curid=7869294. https://en.wikipedia.org/wiki/Chemotherapy-induced_acral_erythema#/media/File:Hand-foot_Syndrome.jpg)

(Figure 51)

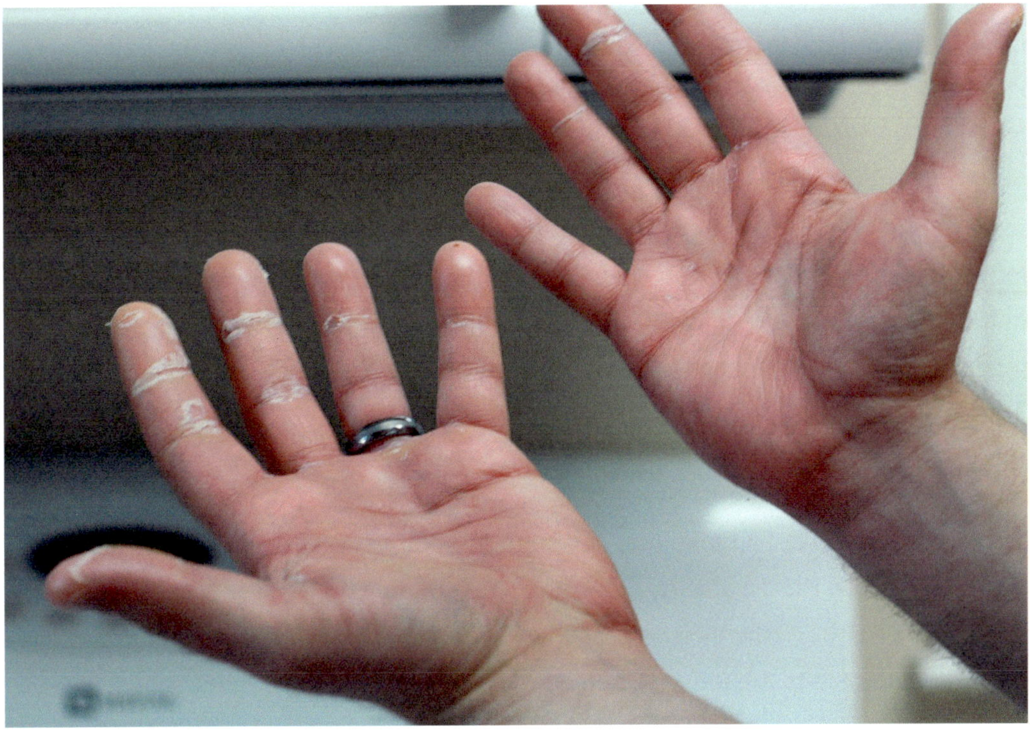

- KEYTRUDA in combination with lenvatinib: *(lenvatinib is a kinase inhibitor that is FDA-approved for the treatment of patients with locally recurrent or metastatic, progressive, radioactive iodine-refractory differentiated thyroid cancer [DTC)]; in combination with everolimus for the treatment of patients with advanced renal cell carcinoma [RCC] following one prior antiangiogenic therapy and for the first-line treatment of patients with unresectable hepatocellular carcinoma [HCC])*

fatigue, hypertension,musculoskeletal pain, diarrhea, decreased appetite, hypothyroidism, nausea, stomatitis, vomiting, decreased weight, abdominal pain, headache, constipation, urinary tract infection, dysphonia, hemorrhagic events, hypomagnesemia, palmar-plantar erythrodysesthesia, dyspnea, cough, and rash.

USE IN SPECIFIC POPULATIONS

Pregnancy risk summary

Based on its mechanism of action, KEYTRUDA can cause fetal harm when administered to a pregnant woman. There are no available human data informing the risk of embryo-fetal toxicity. In animal models, the PD-1/PD-L1 signaling pathway is important in the maintenance of pregnancy through induction of maternal immune tolerance to fetal tissue. Human IgG4 (immunoglobulins) are known to cross the placenta; therefore, pembrolizumab has the potential to be transmitted from the mother to the developing fetus. Advise pregnant women of the potential risk to a fetus. In the U.S. general population, the estimated background risk of major birth defects and miscarriage in clinically recognized pregnancies is 2-4% and 15-20%, respectively.

Animal data

Animal reproduction studies have not been conducted with KEYTRUDA to evaluate its effect on reproduction and fetal development. A literature-based assessment of the effects of the PD-1 pathway on reproduction demonstrated that a central function of the PD-1/PD-L1 pathway is to preserve pregnancy by maintaining maternal immune tolerance to the fetus. Blockade of PD-L1 signaling has been shown in murine models of pregnancy to disrupt tolerance to the fetus and to result in an increase in fetal loss; therefore, potential risks of administering KEYTRUDA during pregnancy include increased rates of abortion or stillbirth. As reported in the literature, there were no malformations related to the blockade of PD-1 signaling in the offspring of these animals; however, immune-mediated disorders occurred in PD-1 knockout mice. Based on its mechanism of action, fetal exposure to pembrolizumab may increase the risk of developing immune-mediated disorders or of altering the normal immune response.

Lactation risk summary

There are no data on the presence of pembrolizumab in either animal or human milk or its effects on the breastfed child or on milk production. Because of the potential for serious adverse reactions in breastfed children, advise women not to breastfeed during treatment with KEYTRUDA and for 4 months after the final dose.

Females and males of reproductive potential pregnancy testing

Verify pregnancy status in females of reproductive potential prior to initiating KEYTRUDA.

Contraception

KEYTRUDA can cause fetal harm when administered to a pregnant woman. Advise females of reproductive potential to use effective contraception during treatment with KEYTRUDA and for at least 4 months following the final dose.

Pediatric use

The safety and effectiveness of KEYTRUDA have been established in pediatric patients with classical Hodgkin Lymphoma (cHL), primary mediastinal large B-cell lymphoma (PMBCL), and microsatellite instability-high (MSI-H) cancer. Use of KEYTRUDA in pediatric patients with cHL, PMBCL, and MSI-H cancers is supported by evidence from adequate and well-controlled studies of KEYTRUDA in adults with additional pharmacokinetic and safety data in pediatric patients. There is limited experience with KEYTRUDA in pediatric patients.

9. Basal cell carcinoma

FDA-approved targeted biologics or specifically designed therapeutic agents for basal cell carcinoma are

Vismodegib/Erivedge

Sonidegib/Odomzo

Cemiplimab-rwlc – please Section 8.1

9.1. Vismodegib/Erivedge

ERIVEDGE™ (vismodegib) capsule for oral use

BOXED WARNING: EMBRYO-FETAL DEATH AND SEVERE BIRTH DEFECTS

ERIVEDGE can result in embryo-fetal death or severe birth defects. Verify pregnancy status prior to initiation of ERIVEDGE. Advise male and female patients of these risks. Advise females of the need for contraception and advise males of the potential risk of ERIVEDGE exposure through semen; decreased appetite, constipation, arthralgias, vomiting, and ageusia *(impairment of taste).* DEFECTS: See full prescribing information for complete boxed warning.

INDICATIONS AND USAGE

ERIVEDGE™ (vismodegib) capsule is a hedgehog pathway inhibitor indicated for the treatment of adults with metastatic basal cell carcinoma, or with locally advanced basal cell carcinoma that has recurred following surgery or who are not candidates for surgery, and who are not candidates for radiation.

DESCRIPTION

Vismodegib is an inhibitor of the hedgehog (Hh) signaling pathway, which is described chemically as 2-Chloro-N-(4-chloro-3-(pyridin-2-yl)phenyl)-4-(methylsulfonyl)benzamide. The molecular formula is C19H14Cl2N2O3S. The molecular weight is 421.30 g/mol and the structural formula is: 189 190 Vismodegib is a crystalline free base with a pKa (pyridinium cation) of 3.8, appearing as a white to tan powder. The solubility of vismodegib is pH dependent with 0.1 μg/mL at pH 7 and 0.99 mg/mL at pH 1. The partition coefficient (log P) is 2.7. 191 192 193 194 Each ERIVEDGE (vismodegib) capsule for oral administration contains 150 mg vismodegib and the 195 following inactive ingredients: microcrystalline cellulose, lactose monohydrate, sodium lauryl 196 sulfate, povidone, sodium starch glycolate, talc, and magnesium stearate (non-bovine). The capsule shell contains gelatin, titanium dioxide, red iron oxide, and black iron oxide. The black printing ink contains shellac and black iron oxide.

MECHANISM OF ACTION

Vismodegib is an inhibitor of the intracellular Hedgehog signalling pathway.

Vismodegib binds to and inhibits Smoothened, a transmembrane protein involved in Hedgehog signal transduction. The Hedgehog signaling pathway is a signaling pathway that transmits information to embryonic cells required for proper cell differentiation. Different parts of the embryo have different concentrations of hedgehog signaling proteins. The pathway also has roles in adult. When Sonic Hedgehog (SHH) reaches its target cell, it binds to the Patched-1 (PTCH1) receptor In the absence of ligand, PTCH1 inhibits Smoothened (SMO), a downstream protein in the pathway.

Figure 52. An overview of Sonic Hedgehog signaling.

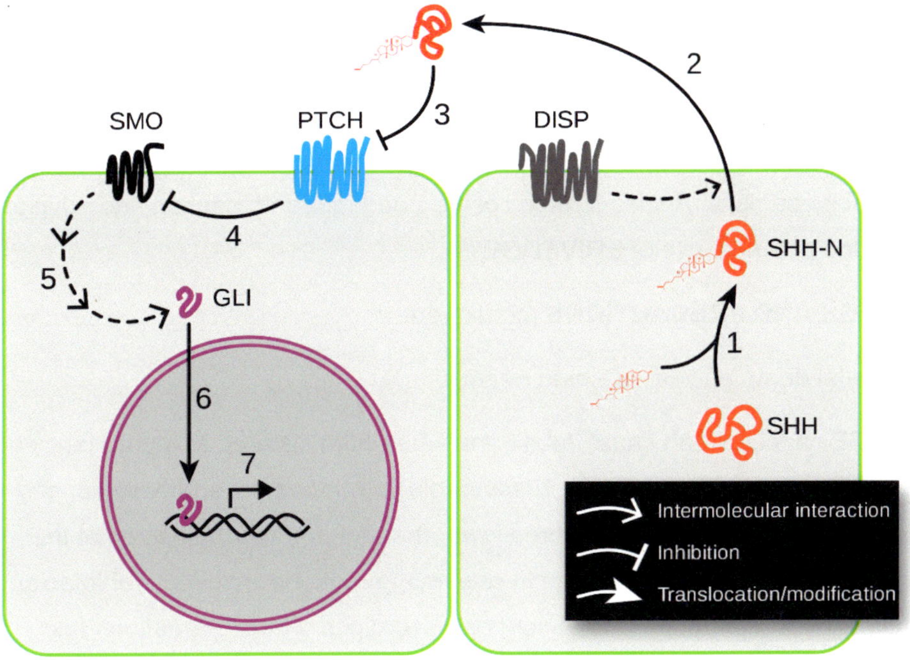

CONTRAINDICATIONS: none.

WARNINGS AND PRECAUTIONS

• Embryo-fetal death and severe birth defects: ERIVEDGE can cause embryo-fetal death or severe birth defects.

• Blood donation: advise patients not to donate blood or blood products while receiving ERIVEDGE and for at least 7 months after the last dose of ERIVEDGE.

ADVERSE REACTIONS

The most common adverse reactions (incidence of ≥ 10%) are muscle spasms, alopecia, dysgeusia, weight loss, fatigue, nausea, diarrhea,

WARNING: EMBRYO-FETAL DEATH AND SEVERE BIRTH DEFECTS, decreased appetite, constipation, arthralgias, vomiting, and ageusia. ERIVEDGE can result in embryo-fetal death or severe birth defects.

Verify pregnancy status prior to initiation of ERIVEDGE. Advise male and female patients of these risks. Advise females of the need for contraception and advise males of the potential risk of ERIVEDGE

WARNINGS AND PRECAUTIONS *(continued)*

Embryo-fetal death and severe birth defects

ERIVEDGE capsules can cause fetal harm when administered to a pregnant woman based on its mechanism of action. Vismodegib is teratogenic, embryotoxic, and fetotoxic in rats at maternal exposures lower than the human exposures at the recommended dose of 150 mg/day. In rats, malformations included craniofacial anomalies, open perineum, and absent or fused digits. Fetal retardations and variations were also observed.

Verify pregnancy status prior to the initiation of ERIVEDGE.

Advise male and female patients of the risks of embryo-fetal death and severe birth defects and the need for contraception during and after treatment. Advise patients to contact their healthcare provider immediately if they suspect they (or, for males, their female partner) may be pregnant. Female and male patients of reproductive potential should be counselled regarding pregnancy prevention and planning. If ERIVEDGE is used during pregnancy or if a patient becomes pregnant while taking (or for a male patient, if his female partner is exposed to) ERIVEDGE, the patient should be apprised of the potential hazard to the fetus. Report immediately exposure to ERIVEDGE during pregnancy to the Genentech Adverse Event Line at 1-888-835-2555.

Encourage women who may have been exposed to ERIVEDGE during pregnancy, either directly or through seminal fluid, to participate in the ERIVEDGE pregnancy pharmacovigilance program by contacting the Genentech Adverse Event Line at 1-888-835-2555.

Blood donation

Advise patients not to donate blood or blood products while receiving ERIVEDGE and for at least 7 months after the last dose of ERIVEDGE

DRUG INTERACTIONS

Effects of other drugs on vismodegib

Drugs that inhibit or induce drug metabolizing enzymes

Vismodegib elimination involves multiple pathways. Vismodegib is predominantly excreted as an unchanged drug. Several minor metabolites are produced by multiple CYP enzymes. Although vismodegib is a substrate of CYP2C9 and CYP3A4 in vitro, CYP inhibition is not predicted to alter vismodegib systemic exposure since similar steady-state plasma vismodegib concentrations were observed in patients in clinical trials concomitantly treated with CYP3A4 inducers (i.e., carbamazepine, modafinil, phenobarbital) and those concomitantly treated with CYP3A4 inhibitors (i.e., erythromycin, fluconazole).

Drugs that inhibit drug transport systems

In vitro studies indicate that vismodegib is a substrate of the efflux transporter P-glycoprotein (P-gp). When ERIVEDGE is co-administered with drugs that inhibit P-gp (e.g. clarithromycin, erythromycin, azithromycin), systemic exposure of vismodegib and incidence of adverse events of ERIVEDGE may be increased.

Drugs that affect gastric pH

Drugs that alter the pH of the upper GI tract (e.g. proton pump inhibitors, H2-receptor antagonists, and antacids) may alter the solubility of vismodegib and reduce its bioavailability. However, no formal clinical study has been conducted to evaluate the effect of gastric pH altering agents on the systemic exposure of vismodegib. Increasing the dose of ERIVEDGE when co-administered with such agents is not likely to compensate for the loss of exposure. When ERIVEDGE is co-administered with a proton pump inhibitor, H2-receptor antagonist or antacid, systemic exposure of vismodegib may be decreased and the effect on efficacy of ERIVEDGE is unknown.

Effects of vismodegib on other drugs

Results of a drug-drug interaction study conducted in cancer patients demonstrated that the systemic exposure of rosiglitazone (a CYP2C8 substrate) or oral contraceptives (ethinyl estradiol and norethindrone) is not altered when either drug is co-administered with vismodegib. In vitro studies indicate that vismodegib is an inhibitor of CYP2C8, CYP2C9, CYP2C19 and the transporter BCRP. Vismodegib does not induce CYP1A2, CYP2B6, or CYP3A4/5 in human hepatocytes.

USE IN SPECIFIC POPULATIONS

Pregnancy

Pregnancy Category D

(Category D pregnancy: there is positive evidence of human fetal risk, but the benefits from use in pregnant women may be acceptable despite the risk (e.g., if the drug is needed in a life-threatening situation or for a serious disease for which safer drugs cannot be used or are ineffective.)

ERIVEDGE capsule can cause fetal harm when administered to a pregnant female based on its mechanism of action. Vismodegib is teratogenic in rats at doses corresponding to an exposure of 20% of the exposure at the recommended human dose (estimated AUC0-24hr steady-state exposure). In rats, malformations included craniofacial anomalies, open perineum, and absent or fused digits. Fetal retardations and variations were also observed. Vismodegib is embryo-lethal in rats at exposures within the range achieved at the recommended human dose. If ERIVEDGE is used during pregnancy, or if the patient becomes pregnant while taking this drug, the patient should be apprised of the potential hazard to the embryo or fetus

In an embryo-fetal developmental toxicity study, pregnant rats were administered oral vismodegib at doses of 10, 60, or 300 mg/kg/day during the period of organogenesis. Pre- and post-implantation loss were increased at doses of ≥ 60 mg/kg/day (approximately ≥ 2 times the systemic exposure (AUC) in patients at the recommended human dose), which included early resorption of 100% of the fetuses. A dose of 10 mg/kg/day (approximately 0.2 times the AUC in patients at the recommended dose) resulted in malformations (including missing and/or fused digits, open perineum and craniofacial anomalies) and retardations or variations (including dilated renal pelvis, dilated ureter, and incompletely or unossified sternal elements, centra of vertebrae, or proximal phalanges and claws).

Nursing mothers

It is not known whether vismodegib is excreted in human breast milk. Because many drugs are excreted in human milk and because of the potential for serious adverse reactions in nursing infants from ERIVEDGE, a decision should be made whether to discontinue nursing or to discontinue the drug, taking into account the importance of the drug to the mother.

Pediatric use

The safety and effectiveness of ERIVEDGE capsule have not been established in pediatric patients. In repeat-dose toxicology studies in rats, administration of oral vismodegib resulted in toxicities in bone and teeth. Effects on bone consisted of closure of the epiphyseal growth plate when oral vismodegib was administered for 26 weeks at ≥ 50 mg/kg/day (approximately ≥ 0.4 times the systemic exposure (AUC) in patients at the recommended human dose). Abnormalities in growing incisor teeth (including degeneration/necrosis of odontoblasts, formation of fluid-filled cysts in the dental pulp, ossification of the root canal, and hemorrhage resulting in breakage or loss of teeth) were observed after administration of oral vismodegib at ≥ 15 mg/kg/day (approximately ≥ 0.2 times the AUC in patients at the recommended human dose).

Geriatric use

Clinical studies of ERIVEDGE capsule did not include sufficient numbers of patients aged 65 and over to determine whether they respond differently from younger patients.

Females of reproductive potential and males

ERIVEDGE capsule can cause harm to the embryo or fetus when administered during pregnancy. Counsel female and male patients regarding pregnancy prevention and planning. Advise patients to contact their healthcare provider immediately if they suspect they (or, for males, their female partner) may be pregnant.

Use in specific populations

Female patients

Determine pregnancy status within 7 days prior to initiation of treatment in females of reproductive potential. For females with a negative pregnancy test, initiate a highly effective form of contraception (failure rate of less than 1%) prior to the first dose. Continue highly effective contraception during therapy and for 7 months after the last dose of ERIVEDGE.

If a patient becomes pregnant while taking ERIVEDGE, or during the 7 months after the last dose of treatment, report the pregnancy to the Genentech Adverse Event Line at 1-888-835-2555. Encourage pregnant females to participate in the ERIVEDGE pregnancy pharmacovigilance program by calling the Genentech Adverse Event Line at 1-888-835-2555.

Counsel pregnant females about the teratogenic risk to the fetus. Amenorrhea has been observed in clinical trials in females of reproductive potential. Reversibility of amenorrhea is unknown.

Male patients

Male patients should use condoms with spermicide, even after a vasectomy, during sexual intercourse with female partners while being treated with ERIVEDGE capsule and for 2 months after the last dose to avoid exposing an embryo or fetus to vismodegib.

Hepatic impairment

The safety and effectiveness of ERIVEDGE capsule have not been established in patients with hepatic impairment.

Renal impairment

The safety and effectiveness of ERIVEDGE capsule have not been established in patients with renal impairment.

OVERDOSAGE

There is no information on overdosage in humans. In clinical trials, ERIVEDGE capsule was administered at 540 mg orally once daily; exposure did not increase between 150 mg and 540 mg daily.

Pharmacokinetics

Absorption

Vismodegib is a highly permeable compound with low aqueous solubility. The single dose absolute bioavailability of vismodegib is 31.8%. Absorption is saturable as evidenced by the lack of dose proportional increase in exposure after a single dose of 270 mg or 540 mg vismodegib.

ERIVEDGE capsules may be taken without regard to meals because the systemic exposure of vismodegib at steady state is not affected by food.

Distribution

The volume of distribution of vismodegib ranges from 16.4 to 26.6 L. Vismodegib plasma protein binding in patients is greater than 99%. Vismodegib binds to both human serum albumin and alpha1-acid glycoprotein (AAG) and binding to AAG is saturable.

Metabolism

Greater than 98% of the total circulating drug-related components are the parent drug. Metabolic pathways of vismodegib in humans include oxidation, glucuronidation, and pyridine ring cleavage. The two most abundant oxidative metabolites recovered in feces are produced in vitro by recombinant CYP2C9 and CYP3A4/5.

Elimination

Vismodegib and its metabolites are eliminated primarily by the hepatic route with 82% of the administered dose recovered in the feces and 4.4% recovered in urine. The estimated elimination half-life (t1/2) of vismodegib is 4 days after continuous once-daily dosing and 12 days after a single dose.

Pharmacokinetics in specific populations

Hepatic impairment

The effect of hepatic impairment on the systemic exposure of vismodegib has not been studied.

Renal Impairment

The effect of renal impairment on the systemic exposure of vismodegib has not been studied.

Population pharmacokinetic analyses showed that weight (range: 41-140 kg), age (range: 26-89 years), creatinine clearance (range: 30 to 80 mL/min), and sex do not have a clinically meaningful influence on the systemic exposure of vismodegib.

Cardiac electrophysiology

In a thorough QTc study in 60 healthy subjects, there was no effect of therapeutic doses of ERIVEDGE on the QTc interval.

9.2. Sonidegib/Odomzo

INDICATIONS AND USAGE

ODOMZO is a hedgehog pathway inhibitor indicated for the treatment of adult patients with

- locally advanced basal cell carcinoma (BCC) that has recurred following surgery or radiation therapy, or
- those who are not candidates for surgery or radiation therapy

DESCRIPTION

ODOMZO (sonidegib) is a **Smoothened** (Smo) antagonist which inhibits the Hedgehog (Hh) signaling pathway. The molecular formula for sonidegib phosphate is C26H26 F3N3O3• 2H3PO4. The molecular weight is 681.49 daltons. The chemical name is N-[6-(cis-2,6-dimethylmorpholin-4-yl)pyridine-3-yl]-2-methyl-4'-(trifluoromethoxy) [1,1'-biphenyl]-3 carboxamide diphosphate. The molecular structure is shown below: sonidegib phosphate is a white to off-white powder. Sonidegib freebase is practically insoluble. Each ODOMZO capsule for oral use contains 200 mg of sonidegib as the freebase (equivalent to 281 mg of diphosphate salt of sonidegib) and the following inactive ingredients: colloidal silicon dioxide, crospovidone, lactose monohydrate, magnesium stearate, poloxamer and sodium lauryl sulfate. The opaque pink hard gelatin capsule shell contains gelatin, red iron oxide, and titanium dioxide. The black printing ink contains ammonium hydroxide, black iron oxide, propylene glycol, and shellac.

MECHANISM OF ACTION

Sonidegib is an inhibitor of the Hedgehog pathway. Sonidegib binds to and inhibits Smoothened, a transmembrane protein involved in Hedgehog signal transduction (See Figure 52).

WARNING

- ODOMZO can cause embryo-fetal death or severe birth defects when administered to a pregnant woman and is embryotoxic, fetotoxic, and teratogenic in animals. Verify the pregnancy status of females of reproductive potential prior to initiating therapy. Advise females of reproductive potential to use effective contraception during treatment with ODOMZO and for at least 20 months after the last dose.
- Advise males of the potential risk of exposure through semen and to use condoms with a pregnant partner or a female partner of reproductive potential during treatment.

EMBRYO-FETAL TOXICITY

CONTRAINDICATIONS: none.

WARNINGS AND PRECAUTIONS

• Blood donation: advise patients not to donate blood or blood products during treatment with ODOMZO and for at least 20 months after the last dose.

• Musculoskeletal adverse reactions: Obtain serum creatine kinase (CK) and creatinine levels prior to initiating therapy, periodically during treatment, and as clinically indicated. Temporary dose interruption or discontinuation of ODOMZO may be required based on the severity of musculoskeletal adverse reactions.

ADVERSE REACTIONS

The most common adverse reactions occurring in ≥10% of patients are muscle spasms, alopecia, dysgeusia, fatigue, nausea, musculoskeletal pain, diarrhea, decreased weight, decreased appetite, myalgia, abdominal pain, headache, pain, vomiting, and pruritus.

To report SUSPECTED ADVERSE REACTIONS, contact Novartis Pharmaceuticals Corporation at 1-888-669-6682 or FDA at 1-800-FDA1088 or www.fda.gov/medwatch.

DRUG INTERACTIONS

• CYP3A inhibitors

Avoid strong CYP3A inhibitors. Avoid long-term (greater than 14 days) use of moderate CYP3A inhibitors.

CYP3A inducers: Avoid strong and moderate CYP3A inducers.

USE IN SPECIFIC POPULATIONS

Lactation

Do not breastfeed during treatment with ODOMZO and for at least 20 months after the last dose.

PRESCRIBING INFORMATION

Dose modifications

Interrupt ODOMZO for

- Severe or intolerable musculoskeletal adverse reactions.
- First occurrence of serum CK elevation between 2.5 and 10 times upper limit of normal (ULN).
- Recurrent serum CK elevation between 2.5 and 5 times ULN. Resume ODOMZO at 200 mg daily upon resolution of clinical signs and symptoms.

Permanently discontinue ODOMZO for

- Serum CK elevation greater than 2.5 times ULN with worsening renal function.
- Serum CK elevation greater than 10 times ULN.
- Recurrent serum CK elevation greater than 5 times ULN.
- Recurrent severe or intolerable musculoskeletal adverse reactions.

Musculoskeletal adverse reactions

Musculoskeletal adverse reactions, which may be accompanied by serum creatine kinase (CK) elevations, occur with ODOMZO and other drugs which inhibit the hedgehog pathway. In a pooled safety analysis of 12 clinical studies involving 571 patients with various advanced cancers treated with ODOMZO at doses ranging from 100 mg to 3000 mg, rhabdomyolysis (defined as serum CK increase of more than ten times the baseline value with a concurrent 1.5-fold or greater increase in serum creatinine above baseline value) occurred in one patient (0.2%) treated with ODOMZO 800 mg. In Study 1, musculoskeletal adverse reactions occurred in 68% (54/79) of patients treated with ODOMZO 200 mg daily with 9% (7/79) reported as Grade 3 or 4. The most frequent manifestations of musculoskeletal adverse reactions reported as an adverse event were muscle spasms (54%), musculoskeletal pain (32%), and myalgia (19%). Increased serum CK laboratory values occurred in 61% (48/79) of patients with 8% (6/79) of patients having Grade 3 or 4 serum CK elevations. Musculoskeletal pain and myalgia usually preceded serum CK elevation. Among patients with Grade 2 or higher CK elevations, the median time to onset was 12.9 weeks (range: 2 to 39 weeks) and the median time to resolution (to ≤ Grade 1) was 12 days (95% CI: 8 to 14 days). ODOMZO was temporarily interrupted in 8% of patients or permanently discontinued in 8% of patients for musculoskeletal adverse reactions. The incidence of musculoskeletal adverse reactions requiring medical intervention (magnesium supplementation, muscle relaxants, and analgesics or narcotics) was 29%, including four patients (5%) who received intravenous hydration or were hospitalized. Obtain baseline serum CK and creatinine levels prior to initiating ODOMZO, periodically during treatment, and as clinically indicated (e.g., if muscle symptoms are reported). Obtain serum creatinine and CK levels at least weekly in patients with musculoskeletal adverse reactions with concurrent serum CK elevation greater than 2.5 times ULN until resolution of clinical signs and symptoms. Depending on the severity of symptoms, temporary dose interruption or discontinuation may be required for musculoskeletal adverse reactions or serum CK elevation.

Advise patients starting therapy with ODOMZO of the risk of muscle-related adverse reactions. Advise patients to report promptly any new unexplained muscle pain, tenderness or weakness occurring during treatment or that persists after discontinuing ODOMZO.

DRUG INTERACTIONS

Effects of other drugs on sonidegib

Strong and moderate CYP3A inhibitors

Avoid concomitant administration of ODOMZO with strong CYP3A inhibitors, including but not limited to saquinavir, telithromycin, ketoconazole, itraconazole, voriconazole, posaconazole and nefazodone.

Avoid concomitant administration of ODOMZO with moderate CYP3A inhibitors, including but not limited to atazanavir, diltiazem, and fluconazole. If a moderate CYP3A inhibitor must be used, administer the moderate CYP3A inhibitor for less than 14 days and monitor closely for adverse reactions particularly musculoskeletal adverse reactions.

Strong and moderate CYP3A inducers

Avoid concomitant administration of ODOMZO with strong and moderate CYP3A inducers, including but not limited to carbamazepine, efavirenz, modafinil, phenobarbital, phenytoin, rifabutin, rifampin and St. John's Wort (Hypericum perforatum).

For further details on drug interaction studies, please see below.

USE IN SPECIFIC POPULATIONS

Pregnancy risk summary

Based on its mechanism of action and data from animal reproduction studies, ODOMZO can cause fetal harm when administered to a pregnant. There are no available data on the use of ODOMZO in pregnant women. In animal reproduction studies, oral administration of sonidegib during organogenesis at doses below the recommended human dose of 200 mg resulted in embryotoxicity, fetotoxicity, and teratogenicity in rabbits. Teratogenic effects observed included severe midline defects, missing digits, and other irreversible malformations. Advise pregnant women of the potential risk to a fetus. Report pregnancies to Novartis Pharmaceuticals Corporation at 1-888-669-6682. The background risk of major birth defects and miscarriage for the indicated population is unknown; however, the background risk in the U.S. general population of major birth defects is 2-4% and of miscarriage is 15-20% of clinically recognized pregnancies.

Data

Animal data

Daily oral administration of sonidegib to pregnant rabbits resulted in abortion, complete resorption of fetuses, or severe malformations at ≥ 5 mg/kg/day (approximately 0.05 times the recommended human dose based on AUC). Teratogenic effects included vertebral, distal limb and digit malformations, severe craniofacial malformations, and other severe midline defects. Skeletal variations were observed when maternal exposure to sonidegib was below the limit of detection.

Lactation

No data are available regarding the presence of sonidegib in human milk, the effects of the drug on the breast fed infant, or the effects of the drug on milk production.

Because of the potential for serious adverse reactions in breastfed infants from sonidegib, advise a nursing woman not to breastfeed during treatment with ODOMZO and for 20 months after the last dose.

Females and males of reproductive potential

Based on its mechanism of action and animal data, ODOMZO can cause fetal harm when administered to a pregnant woman.

Pregnancy testing

Verify the pregnancy status of females of reproductive potential prior to initiating ODOMZO treatment.

Contraception

Females

Advise females of reproductive potential to use effective contraception during treatment with ODOMZO and for at least 20 months after the last dose.

Males

It is not known if sonidegib is present in semen. Advise male patients to use condoms, even after a vasectomy, to avoid potential drug exposure to pregnant partners and female partners of reproductive potential during treatment with ODOMZO and for at least 8 months after the last dose. Advise males not to donate semen during treatment with ODOMZO and for at least 8 months after the last dose.

Infertility

Based on findings from animal studies, female fertility may be compromised with ODOMZO

Pediatric use

The safety and effectiveness of ODOMZO have not been established in pediatric patients.

Juvenile animal data

In a 5-week juvenile rat toxicology study, effects of sonidegib were observed in bone, teeth, reproductive tissues, and nerves at doses ≥10 mg/kg/day (approximately 1.2

times the recommended human dose based on AUC). Bone findings included thinning/closure of bone growth plate, decreased bone length and width, and hyperostosis. Findings in teeth included missing or fractured teeth, and atrophy. Reproductive tissue toxicity was evidenced by atrophy of testes, ovaries, and uterus, partial development of the prostate gland and seminal vesicles, and inflammation and aspermia of the epididymis. Nerve degeneration was also noted.

Geriatric use

Of the 229 patients who received ODOMZO (79 patients receiving 200 mg daily and 150 patients receiving 800 mg daily) in Study 1, 54% were 65 years and older, while 28% were 75 years and older. No overall differences in effectiveness were observed between these patients and younger patients. There was a higher incidence of serious adverse events, Grade 3 and 4 adverse events, and adverse events requiring dose interruption or discontinuation in patients ≥65 years compared with younger patients; this was not attributable to an increase in any specific adverse event.

OVERDOSAGE

There are no recommendations regarding management of overdosage.

Pharmacodynamics Cardiac Electrophysiology At a dose of 800 mg once daily, sonidegib does not prolong the QTc interval.

Pharmacokinetics

Absorption

Less than 10% of an oral dose of ODOMZO is absorbed. Following the administration of a single ODOMZO dose (100 mg to 3000 mg) under fasted conditions in patients with cancer, the median time-to-peak concentration (Tmax) was 2 to 4 hours. Sonidegib exhibited dose-proportional increases in the area under the curve (AUC) and the maximal concentration (Cmax) over the dose range of 100 mg to 400 mg, but less than dose-proportional increases at doses greater than 400 mg. Steady-state was reached approximately 4 months after starting ODOMZO and the estimated accumulation at steady-state was 19-fold. Following a dose of 200 mg once daily, the estimated mean steady-state Cmax is 1030 ng/mL, AUC0-24h is 22 µg*h/mL and minimal concentration (Cmin) is 890 ng/mL. A high-fat meal (approximately 1000 calories with 50% of calories from fat) increased exposure to sonidegib (geometric mean AUCinf and Cmax) by 7.4- to 7.8-fold.

Distribution

The estimated apparent steady-state volume of distribution (Vss/F) was 9,166 L. Sonidegib was greater than 97% bound to human plasma proteins in vitro and the binding was concentration independent. In vitro studies suggested that sonidegib is not a substrate of P-glycoprotein, MRP2 or BCRP.

Elimination

The elimination half-life (t1/2) of sonidegib estimated from population pharmacokinetic (PK) modeling was approximately 28 days.

Metabolism

Sonidegib is primarily metabolized by CYP3A. The main circulating compound was unchanged sonidegib (36% of circulating radioactivity).

Excretion

Sonidegib and its metabolites are eliminated primarily by the hepatic route. Of the absorbed dose, approximately 70% was eliminated in the feces and 30% was eliminated in the urine. Unchanged sonidegib was not detectable in the urine.

Specific populations

Hepatic Impairment *(see Appendix X for Child-Pugh classification of hepatic function impairment)*

Mild (Child-Pugh class A), moderate (Child-Pugh class B), or severe (Child-Pugh class C) hepatic impairment had no clinically meaningful effect on sonidegib exposure as compared to subjects with normal hepatic function.

Renal Impairment

Mild (CLcr 60 to 89 mL/min) and moderate (CLcr 30 to 59 mL/min) renal impairment had no effect on sonidegib steadystate exposure as compared to patients with normal renal function (CLcr ≥90 mL/min).

Age, Sex, Weight and Race Age, body weight, or sex had no clinically meaningful effect on sonidegib steady-state exposure. A cross study comparison suggests that geometric mean AUCinf of sonidegib is 1.7-fold higher in Japanese healthy subjects compared to Western healthy subjects (Whites and Blacks) following a single 200 mg dose of ODOMZO.

Drug interaction studies

Effects of CYP3A Inhibitors on Sonidegib

Strong CYP3A inhibitors

The geometric mean sonidegib AUC0-10d increased by 2.2-fold and the Cmax increased by 1.5 fold when ODOMZO at a dose of 800 mg was taken with ketoconazole compared to ODOMZO alone. The geometric mean sonidegib steady-state AUC0-24h would similarly increase in cancer patients taking ODOMZO 200 mg once daily when co-administered with a strong CYP3A inhibitor for 14 days.

Moderate CYP3A inhibitors

The geometric mean sonidegib steady-state AUC0-24h would increase 1.8-fold when ODOMZO 200 mg once daily is co-administered with a moderate CYP3A inhibitor (erythromycin) for 14 days and would increase 2.8-fold when ODOMZO 200 mg once daily is co-administered with a moderate CYP3A inhibitor (erythromycin) for 4 months.

Effects of CYP3A Inducers on Sonidegib

Strong CYP3A inducers

The geometric mean sonidegib AUC0-10d decreased by 72% and the Cmax decreased by 54% when ODOMZO at a dose of 800 mg was taken with rifampicin compared to ODOMZO alone.

Moderate CYP3A inducer

Geometric mean sonidegib steady-state AUC0-24h would decrease 56% in cancer patients taking ODOMZO 200 mg once daily when co-administered with a moderate CYP3A inducer (efavirenz) for 14 days and would decrease 69% when co-administered with a moderate CYP3A inducer (efavirenz) for 4 months

Effect of Sonidegib on Cytochrome P450 enzymes and transporters

In vitro studies suggested that sonidegib inhibits CYP2B6 and CYP2C9 and it does not induce CYP1A2, CYP2B6 or CYP3A expression or activity. In vitro studies suggested that sonidegib inhibits BCRP, but not P-glycoprotein, MRP2, OATP1B1, OATP1B3, OAT1, OAT3, OCT1 or OCT2.

Effect of acid reducing agents on sonidegib

No clinically meaningful effect on sonidegib exposure was observed when ODOMZO at a dose of 200 mg was co-administered with esomeprazole, a proton pump inhibitor.

10. Merkel cell carcinoma

10.1. FDA-approved medications for Merkel cell carcinoma are

Avelumab

Pembrolizumab (please see Section X)

10.2. Avelumab

FDA-approved targeted biologics for Merkel cell carcinoma are

Avelumab/BAVENCIO®

Pembolizumab/Keytruda - Please see Section 8.3 for details.

Avelumab

DESCRIPTION

Avelumab is a programmed death ligand1 (PD-L1) blocking antibody. Avelumab is a human IgG1 lambda monoclonal antibody produced in Chinese hamster ovary cells and has a molecular weight of approximately 147 kDa. BAVENCIO (avelumab) Injection for intravenous use is a sterile, preservative-free, nonpyrogenic, clear, colorless to slightly yellow solution. Each single-dose vial contains 200 mg avelumab in 10 mL (20 mg/mL). Each mL contains 20 mg avelumab, D-mannitol (51 mg), glacial acetic acid (0.6 mg), polysorbate 20 (0.5 mg), sodium hydroxide (0.3 mg), and Water for Injection. The pH range of the solution is 5.0 – 5.6.

MECHANISM OF ACTION

PD-L1 may be expressed on tumor cells and tumor-infiltrating immune cells and can contribute to the inhibition of the anti-tumor immune response in the tumor microenvironment. Binding of PD-L1 to the PD-1 and B7.1 receptors found on T cells and antigen-presenting cells suppresses cytotoxic T cell activity, T cell proliferation, and cytokine production. Avelumab binds PD-L1 and blocks the interaction between PD-L1 and its receptors PD-1 and B7.1. This interaction releases the inhibitory effects of PD-L1 on the immune response resulting in the restoration of immune responses, including anti-tumor immune responses. Avelumab has also been shown to induce antibody-dependent cell-mediated cytotoxicity (ADCC) in vitro. In syngeneic mouse tumor models, blocking PD-L1 activity resulted in decreased tumor growth

INDICATIONS AND USAGE

Metastatic Merkel Cell Carcinoma

BAVENCIO (avelumab) is indicated for the treatment of adults and pediatric patients 12 years and older with metastatic Merkel cell carcinoma (MCC). This indication is approved under accelerated approval based on tumor response rate and duration of response. Continued approval for this indication may be contingent upon verification and description of clinical benefit in confirmatory trials

(Bavencio is also FDA-approved for the treatment of advanced urothelial cancer and advanced renal cancer but only its application for Merkel cell carcinoma is dealt with in this book).

WARNINGS AND PRECAUTIONS

Immune-mediated pneumonitis *(please see Section X for images)*

BAVENCIO can cause immune-mediated pneumonitis, including fatal cases. Monitor patients for signs and symptoms of pneumonitis and evaluate patients with suspected pneumonitis with radiographic imaging. Administer corticosteroids (initial dose of 1 to 2 mg/kg/day prednisone or equivalent, followed by a corticosteroid taper) for Grade 2 or greater pneumonitis. Withhold BAVENCIO for moderate (Grade

2) pneumonitis, and permanently discontinue for severe (Grade 3), life-threatening (Grade 4), or recurrent moderate (Grade 2) pneumonitis.

Pneumonitis occurred in 1.2% of patients receiving BAVENCIO including one (0.1%) patient with Grade 5, one (0.1%) with Grade 4, and five (0.3%) with Grade 3 pneumonitis. Immune-mediated pneumonitis led to permanent discontinuation of BAVENCIO in 0.3% of patients. Among the 21 patients with immune-mediated pneumonitis, the median time to onset was 2.5 months (range: 3 days to 11 months) and the median duration of pneumonitis was 7 weeks (range: 4 days to 4+ months). All 21 patients were treated with systemic corticosteroids; 17 (81%) of the 21 patients received high-dose corticosteroids for a median of 8 days (range: 1 day to 2.3 months).

Resolution of pneumonitis occurred in 12 (57%) of the 21 patients at the time of data cut-off.

Hepatotoxicity and immune-mediated hepatitis

BAVENCIO can cause immune-mediated hepatitis including fatal cases. Monitor patients for abnormal liver tests prior to and periodically during treatment. Administer corticosteroids (initial dose of 1 to 2 mg/kg/day prednisone or equivalent, followed by a corticosteroid taper) for Grade 2 or greater hepatitis. Withhold BAVENCIO for moderate (Grade 2) immune-mediated hepatitis until resolution and permanently discontinue for severe (Grade 3) or life-threatening (Grade 4) immune-mediated hepatitis

BAVENCIO as a single agent

Immune-mediated hepatitis occurred in 0.9% of patients receiving BAVENCIO including two (0.1%) patients with Grade 2 and 11 (0.6 %) patients with Grade 3 immune-mediated hepatitis. Immune-mediated hepatitis led to permanent discontinuation of BAVENCIO in 0.5% of patients. Among the 16 patients with immune-mediated hepatitis, the median time to onset was 3.2 months (range: 1 week to 15 months), and the median duration of hepatitis was 2.5 months (range: 1 day to 7.4+ months). All 16 patients were treated with corticosteroids; 15 (94%) of the 16 patients received high-dose corticosteroids for a median of 14 days (range: 1

day to 2.5 months). Resolution of hepatitis occurred in nine (56%) of the 16 patients at the time of data cut-off.

BAVENCIO with Axitinib *(axitinib is a small molecule tyrosine kinase inhibitor which is FDA-approved for advanced renal cell carcinoma [RCC])*

BAVENCIO in combination with axitinib can cause hepatotoxicity with higher than expected frequencies of Grade 3 and 4 ALT and AST elevation. Consider more frequent monitoring of liver enzymes as compared to when the drugs are used as monotherapy. Withhold BAVENCIO and axitinib for moderate (Grade 2) hepatotoxicity and permanently discontinue the combination for severe or life-threatening (Grade 3 or 4) hepatotoxicity. Administer corticosteroids as needed. In patients treated with BAVENCIO in combination with axitinib in the advanced RCC trials, Grades 3 and 4 increased ALT and increased AST were reported in 9% and 7% of patients, respectively. In patients with ALT ≥ 3 times ULN (Grades 2-4, n=82), ALT resolved to Grades 0-1 in 92%. Among the 73 patients who were rechallenged with either BAVENCIO (59%) or axitinib (85%) monotherapy or with both (55%), 66% had no recurrence of ALT ≥ 3 times ULN. Immune-mediated hepatitis was reported in 7% of patients including 4.9% with Grade 3 or 4 immune-mediated hepatitis. Hepatotoxicity led to permanent discontinuation in 6.5% and immune-mediated hepatitis led to permanent discontinuation of either BAVENCIO or axitinib in 5.3% of patients. Among the 35 patients with immune-mediated hepatitis, the median time to onset was 2.8 months (range: 2.1 weeks to 14.5 months) and the median duration of hepatitis was 15 days (range: 2 days to 9 months). Thirty-four patients were treated with corticosteroids and one patient was treated with a non-steroidal immunosuppressant; 33 patients received high-dose corticosteroids for a median of 21 days (range: 4 days to 3 months). Resolution of hepatitis occurred in 31 of the 35 patients at the time of data cut-off.

Immune-mediated colitis (see Section X for images)

BAVENCIO can cause immune-mediated colitis.

Monitor patients for signs and symptoms of colitis. Administer corticosteroids (initial dose of 1 to 2 mg/kg/day prednisone or equivalent followed by a corticosteroid taper) for Grade 2 or greater colitis. Withhold BAVENCIO for moderate or severe (Grade 2 or 3) colitis until resolution. Permanently discontinue BAVENCIO for life-threatening

(Grade 4) or for recurrent (Grade 3) colitis upon reinitiation of BAVENCIO. Immune-mediated colitis occurred in 1.5% of patients receiving BAVENCIO including seven (0.4%) patients with Grade 3 colitis. Immune-mediated colitis led to permanent discontinuation of BAVENCIO in 0.5% of patients. Among the 26 patients with immune-mediated colitis, the median time to onset was 2.1 months (range: 2 days to 11 months) and the median duration of colitis was 6 weeks (range: 1 day to 14+ months). All 26 patients were treated with corticosteroids; 15 (58%) of the 26 patients received high-dose corticosteroids for a median of 19 days (range: 1 day to 2.3 months). Resolution of colitis occurred in 18 (70%) of the patients at the time of data cut-off.

Immune-mediated endocrinopathies

BAVENCIO can cause immune-mediated endocrinopathies.

Adrenal insufficiency

Monitor patients for signs and symptoms of adrenal insufficiency during and after treatment. Administer corticosteroids as appropriate for adrenal insufficiency. Withhold BAVENCIO for severe (Grade 3) or life-threatening (Grade 4) adrenal insufficiency. Adrenal insufficiency occurred in 0.5% of patients receiving BAVENCIO including one patient (0.1%) with Grade 3 adrenal insufficiency. Immune-mediated adrenal insufficiency led to permanent discontinuation of BAVENCIO in 0.1% of patients. Among the 8 patients with immune-mediated adrenal insufficiency, the median time to onset was 2.5 months (range: 1 day to 8 months). All eight patients were treated with corticosteroids; four (50%) of the eight patients received high-dose corticosteroids for a median of 1 day (range: 1 day to 24 days).

Thyroid Disorders (Hypothyroidism/Hyperthyroidism)

BAVENCIO can cause immune-mediated thyroid disorders. Thyroid disorders can occur at any time during treatment. Monitor patients for changes in thyroid function at the start of treatment, periodically during treatment, and as indicated based on clinical evaluation. Manage hypothyroidism with hormone-replacement therapy. Initiate medical management for control of hyperthyroidism. Withhold BAVENCIO for severe (Grade 3) or life-threatening (Grade 4) thyroid disorders.

Immune-mediated thyroid disorders occurred in 6% of patients receiving BAVENCIO including 3 (0.2%) Grade 3 immune-mediated thyroid disorders. Immune-mediated thyroid disorders led to discontinuation of BAVENCIO in 0.1% of patients. Hypothyroidism occurred in 90 (5%) patients; hyperthyroidism in seven (0.4%) patients; and thyroiditis in four (0.2%) patients treated with BAVENCIO. Among the 98 patients with immune-mediated thyroid disorders, the median time to onset was 2.8 months (range: 2 weeks to 13 months) and the median duration was not estimable (range: 6 days to more than 26 months). Immune-mediated thyroid disorders resolved in seven (7%) of the 98 patients.

Type 1 Diabetes mellitus *(please see Section X for images)*

BAVENCIO can cause type 1 diabetes mellitus, including diabetic ketoacidosis. Monitor patients for hyperglycemia or other signs and symptoms of diabetes. Withhold BAVENCIO and administer anti-hyperglycemics or insulin in patients with severe or life-threatening (Grade ≥ 3) hyperglycemia. Resume treatment with BAVENCIO when metabolic control is achieved on insulin replacement or anti-hyperglycemics.Type 1 diabetes mellitus without an alternative etiology occurred in 0.1% of patients including two cases of Grade 3 hyperglycemia that led to permanent discontinuation of BAVENCIO.

Immune-mediated nephritis and renal dysfunction

BAVENCIO can cause immune-mediated nephritis. Monitor patients for elevated serum creatinine prior to and periodically during treatment. Administer corticosteroids (initial dose of 1 to 2 mg/kg/day prednisone or equivalent followed by a corticosteroid taper) for Grade 2 or greater nephritis. Withhold BAVENCIO for moderate (Grade 2) or severe (Grade 3) nephritis until resolution to ≤ Grade 1. Permanently discontinue BAVENCIO for life-threatening (Grade 4) nephritis.

Immune-mediated nephritis occurred in 0.1% of patients receiving BAVENCIO; BAVENCIO was permanently discontinued in this patient.

Other immune-mediated adverse reactions

BAVENCIO can result in severe and fatal immune-mediated adverse reactions. These immune-mediated reactions may involve any organ system. Most immune-mediated reactions initially manifest during treatment with BAVENCIO; however, immune-mediated adverse reactions can occur after discontinuation of BAVENCIO. For suspected immune-mediated adverse reactions, evaluate to confirm or rule out an immune-mediated adverse reaction and to exclude other causes. Depending upon the severity of the adverse reaction, withhold or permanently discontinue BAVENCIO, administer high dose corticosteroids, and if appropriate, initiate hormone replacement therapy. Upon improvement to Grade 1 or less, initiate corticosteroid taper. Resume BAVENCIO when the immune-mediated adverse reaction remains at Grade 1 or less following corticosteroid taper. Permanently discontinue BAVENCIO for any severe (Grade 3) immune-mediated adverse reaction that recurs and for any life-threatening immune-mediated adverse reaction.

The following clinically significant, immune-mediated adverse reactions occurred at an incidence of less than 1% of patients who received BAVENCIO as a single agent or in 489 patients who received BAVENCIO in combination with axitinib: **immune-mediated myocarditis** including fatal cases, pancreatitis including fatal cases, immune-mediated myositis, **psoriasis, arthritis, exfoliative dermatitis, erythema multiforme, pemphigoid, hypopituitarism, uveitis, Guillain-Barré syndrome**, and **systemic inflammatory response**. The following clinically significant, immune-mediated adverse reactions have been reported with other products in this class: bullous dermatitis, Stevens Johnson Syndrome (SJS)/toxic epidermal necrolysis (TEN), rhabdomyolysis, myasthenia gravis, histiocytic necrotizing lymphadenitis, demyelination, vasculitis, hemolytic anemia, hypophysitis, iritis, and encephalitis.

Infusion-related reactions

BAVENCIO can cause severe or life-threatening infusion-related reactions. Premedicate with antihistamine and acetaminophen prior to the first 4 infusions. Monitor patients for signs and symptoms of infusion-related reactions including pyrexia, chills, flushing, hypotension, dyspnea, wheezing, back pain, abdominal pain, and urticaria. Interrupt or slow the rate of infusion for mild or moderate infusion-related reactions. Stop the infusion and permanently discontinue BAVENCIO for severe (Grade 3) or lifethreatening (Grade 4) infusion-related reactions. Infusion-related reactions occurred in 25% of patients treated with BAVENCIO including three (0.2%) Grade 4 and nine (0.5%) Grade 3 infusion-related reactions. Ninety-three percent of patients received premedication with antihistamine and acetaminophen.

Eleven (92%) of the 12 patients with Grade ≥ 3 reactions were treated with intravenous corticosteroids. Fourteen percent of patients had infusion-related reactions that occurred after the BAVENCIO infusion was completed.

Major adverse cardiovascular events (MACE)

BAVENCIO in combination with axitinib can cause severe and fatal cardiovascular events. Consider baseline and periodic evaluations of left ventricular ejection fraction. Monitor for signs and symptoms of cardiovascular events. Optimize management of cardiovascular risk factors, such as hypertension, diabetes, or dyslipidemia. Discontinue BAVENCIO and axitinib for Grade 3-4 cardiovascular events. MACE occurred in 7% of patients with advanced RCC treated with BAVENCIO in combination with axitinib compared to 3.4% treated with sunitinib in a randomized trial, JAVELIN Renal 101. These events included death due to cardiac events (1.4%), Grade 3-4 myocardial infarction (2.8%), and Grade 3-4 congestive heart failure (1.8%). Median time to onset of MACE was 4.2 months (range: 2 days to 24.5 months).

Embryo-fetal toxicity

Based on its mechanism of action, BAVENCIO can cause fetal harm when administered to a pregnant woman. Animal studies have demonstrated that inhibition of the PD-1/PD-L1 pathway can lead to increased risk of immune-mediated rejection of the developing fetus resulting in fetal death. If this drug is used during pregnancy, or if the patient becomes pregnant while taking BAVENCIO, inform the patient of the potential risk to a fetus. Advise females of childbearing potential to use effective contraception during treatment with BAVENCIO and for at least one month after the last dose of BAVENCIO.

Immunogenicity

As with all therapeutic proteins, there is potential for immunogenicity. The detection of antibody formation is highly dependent on the sensitivity and specificity of the assay. Additionally, the observed incidence of antibody (including neutralizing antibody) positivity in an assay may be influenced by several factors including assay methodology, sample handling, timing of sample collection, concomitant medications, and underlying disease. For these reasons, comparison of the incidence of antibodies to avelumab in the studies described below with the incidence of antibodies in other studies or to other products may be misleading. Of the 1738 patients treated with BAVENCIO 10 mg/kg as an intravenous infusion every 2 weeks, 1558 were evaluable for treatment-emergent anti-drug antibodies (ADA) and 64 (4.1%) tested positive. The development of treatment-emergent ADA against avelumab did not appear to alter the pharmacokinetic profile or risk of infusion-related reactions. Of the 480 patients treated with BAVENCIO 10 mg/kg as an intravenous infusion every 2 weeks in combination with axitinib 5 mg twice daily, 453 were evaluable for treatment-emergent antidrug antibodies (ADA) and 66 (15%) tested positive. A new ADA method with improved sensitivity was used in the RCC population. Patients who tested positive for treatment-emergent ADA had decreased systemic BAVENCIO exposure. The development of treatment-emergent ADA against avelumab did not appear to alter the risk of infusion-related reactions.

USE IN SPECIFIC POPULATIONS

Pregnancy risk summary

Based on its mechanism of action, BAVENCIO can cause fetal harm when administered to a pregnant woman. There are no available data on the use of BAVENCIO in pregnant women. Animal studies have demonstrated that inhibition of the PD-1/PD-L1 pathway can lead to increased risk of immune-mediated rejection of the developing fetus resulting in fetal death [see Data]. Human IgG1 immunoglobulins (IgG1) are known to cross the placenta. Therefore, BAVENCIO has the potential to be transmitted from the mother to the developing fetus. If this drug is used during pregnancy, or if the patient becomes pregnant while taking this drug, advise the patient of the potential risk to a fetus.

In the U.S. general population, the estimated background risk of major birth defects and miscarriage in clinically recognized pregnancies is 2% to 4% and 15% to 20%, respectively.

Data

Animal Data

Animal reproduction studies have not been conducted with BAVENCIO to evaluate its effect on reproduction and fetal development. A central function of the PD-1/PD-

L1 pathway is to preserve pregnancy by maintaining maternal immune tolerance to the fetus. In murine models of pregnancy, blockade of PD-L1 signaling has been shown to disrupt tolerance to the fetus and to result in an increase in fetal loss; therefore, potential risks of administering BAVENCIO during pregnancy include increased rates of abortion or stillbirth. As reported in the literature, there were no malformations related to the blockade of PD-1/PD-L1 signaling in the offspring of these animals; however, immune-mediated disorders occurred in PD-1 and PD-L1 knockout mice. Based on its mechanism of action, fetal exposure to BAVENCIO may increase the risk of developing immune-related disorders or altering the normal immune response.

Lactation risk summary

There is no information regarding the presence of avelumab in human milk, the effects on the breastfed infant, or the effects on milk production. Since many drugs including antibodies are excreted in human milk, advise a lactating woman not to breastfeed during treatment and for at least one month after the last dose of BAVENCIO due to the potential for serious adverse reactions in breastfed infants.

Females and males of reproductive potential

Contraception

Based on its mechanism of action, BAVENCIO can cause fetal harm when administered to a pregnant woman. Advise females of reproductive potential to use effective contraception during treatment with BAVENCIO and for at least 1 month after the last dose of BAVENCIO.

Pediatric use

The safety and effectiveness of BAVENCIO have been established in pediatric patients aged 12 years and older for metastatic MCC. Use of BAVENCIO in this age group is supported by evidence from adequate and well-controlled studies of BAVENCIO in adults with additional population pharmacokinetic data demonstrating that age and body weight had no clinically meaningful effect on the steady state exposure of avelumab, that drug exposure is generally similar between adults and pediatric patients age 12 years and older for monoclonal antibodies, and that the course of MCC is sufficiently similar in adult and pediatric patients to allow extrapolation of data in adults to pediatric patients. The recommended dose in pediatric patients 12 years of age or greater is the same as that in adults.

Clinical pharmacology and clinical studies

Safety and effectiveness of BAVENCIO have not been established in pediatric patients less than 12 years of age.

Geriatric use

Clinical studies of BAVENCIO in MCC did not include sufficient numbers of patients aged 65 and over to determine whether they respond differently from younger patients.

Pharmacokinetics

Avelumab pharmacokinetics (PK) was assessed using a population PK approach for both single agent BAVENCIO and BAVENCIO in combination with axitinib. There are no expected clinically meaningful differences in exposure of avelumab administered every 2 weeks at 800 mg or 10 mg/kg in both settings.

BAVENCIO as a single agent

The pharmacokinetics of avelumab as a single agent was studied in 1629 patients who received doses ranging from 1 to 20 mg/kg every 2 weeks. The data showed that the exposure of avelumab increased dose-proportionally in the dose range of 10 to 20 mg/kg every 2 weeks. Steady-state concentrations of avelumab were reached after approximately 4 to 6 weeks (2 to 3 cycles) of repeated dosing, and the systemic accumulation was approximately 1.25-fold. The geometric mean volume of distribution at steady state for a subject receiving 10 mg/kg was 4.72 L.

The primary elimination mechanism of avelumab is proteolytic degradation. Based on population pharmacokinetic analyses in patients with solid tumors, the total systemic clearance was 0.59 L/day and the terminal half-life was 6.1 days in patients receiving 10 mg/kg. In a post hoc analysis, avelumab clearance was found to decrease over time in patients with MCC, with a mean maximal reduction (% coefficient of variation [CV%]) from baseline value of approximately 32.1% (36.2%), which is not considered clinically important. There was no evidence to suggest a change of avelumab clearance over time in patients with UC.

BAVENCIO with axitinib

When BAVENCIO 10 mg/kg was administered in combination with axitinib 5 mg, the respective exposures of avelumab and axitinib were comparable to the single agents.

Specific populations

Body weight was positively correlated with total systemic clearance in population pharmacokinetic analyses. No clinically meaningful differences in pharmacokinetics were observed in the clearance of avelumab based on age; sex; race; PD-L1 status; tumor burden; mild [calculated creatinine clearance (CLcr) 60 to 89 mL/min, n=623 as estimated by the Cockcroft-Gault formula], moderate [CLcr 30 to 59 mL/min, n=320], or severe [CLcr 15 to 29 mL/min, n=4] renal impairment; and mild [bilirubin less than or equal to ULN and AST greater than ULN or bilirubin between 1 and 1.5 times ULN, n=217] or moderate [bilirubin between 1.5 and 3 times ULN, n=4] hepatic impairment. There are limited data from patients with severe hepatic impairment [bilirubin greater than 3 times ULN, n=1], and the effect of severe hepatic impairment on the pharmacokinetics of avelumab is unknown.

CONCLUSIONS

Cutaneous squamous cell carcinoma (cSCC)

For **localized disease**, wide surgical resection is the appropriate treatment if possible. Topical fluoruracil is valuable for large lesions (>3 cm in diameter) and in situations in which postoperative healing is compromised, such as lesions that involve the lower extremity in older adult patients or patients with venous stasis disease.

For **advanced or metastatic cSCC** not amenable to loco-regional treatment, administration of an immune checkpoint inhibitor, either cemiplimab or pembrolizumab, is recommended. However, as of March 2021, the Pharmaceutical Benefits Advisory Committee of Australia (PBAC) did **not** recommend cemiplimab for the treatment of patients with metastatic or locally advanced cutaneous squamous cell carcinoma (mCSCC or laCSCC). It appears that pembolizumab is also **not** PBAC-approved for locally advanced cSCC not curable with surgery or radiation therapy, although the USA FDA expanded its approval for pembrolizumab to include patients with locally advanced cSCC not curable with surgery or radiation therapy as of September 2021.

If the disease progresses despite the use of a checkpoint inhibitor, or if the patient was ineligible for the use of a checkpoint inhibitor, chemotherapy with carboplatin and paclitaxel is the last option other than the use of the EGFR inhibitor cetuximab. As far as I can determine, cetuximab is TGA-approved in Australia for sqamous cell carcinoma of the head and neck but **not** for cutaneous SCC.

Basal cell carcinomaof the skin (BCC)

For localized disease, wide surgical resection is the appropriate treatment if possible. Topical imiquimod is a topical immune response modifier approved for the treatment of superficial basal cell carcinoma. Its antitumor effects are thought to be mediated by the stimulation of local cytokine production, cell-mediated immunity, and, possibly, the promotion of apoptosis

For locally advanced basal cell carcinoma that is not amenable to surgery or radiation, either of the inhibitors of the intracellular Hedgehog signalling pathway, vismodegib or sonidegib, may be used. For metastatic BCC vismodegib is preferred to sonidegib.

For patients with locally advanced or metastatic BCCs who have progressed on, or are intolerant of the use of vismodegib or sonidegib, the checkpoint inhibitor cemiplimab is indicated. However, as of November 2020 the PBAC did **not** recommend cemiplimab for the treatment of patients with metastatic or locally advanced cutaneous squamous cell carcinoma (mCSCC or laCSCC) who are not candidates for curative surgery or curative radiation.

Merkel cell carcinoma (MCC)

For a person with a biopsy-confirmed cutaneous MCC, the initial evaluation should focus on determining whether there is clinical evidence of lymph node involvement or distant metastasis. Baseline determination of Merkel virus oncoprotein antibody titer can assist with prognosis and subsequent detection of recurrent disease. Imaging studies are important because of the metastatic potential of this cancer. For people without evidence of regional lymph node or distant metastases, sentinel lymph node (SLN) mapping and biopy are indicated to rule out occult disease. For those with a positive SLN biopsy, evaluation for occult metastatic disease is indicated. If no distant metastatic disease is detected, treatment of the regional lymph node area is indicated with either nodal dissection or radiation therapy (RT). Adjuvant RT is offered after node dissection for multiple nodal involvement or extranodal extension.

For those without regional lymphatic or distant metastases, resection of the primary lesion with a margin of 1 to 2 cm should be undertaken. This should be followed by adjuvant radiation if high risk factors are present. These include a primary tumor ≥1 cm in maximum dimension, positive or limited surgical resection margins, lymphovascular invasion, or an immunocompromised host.

Radiotherapy (RT) is an alternative to surgery for patients who are not surgical candidates or for those in whom wide excision of the primary tumor is not feasible,

Patients with metastatic disease should receive nitial treatment with a programmed cell death ligand 1 (PD-L1)-blocking agent (avelumab) or programmed cell death protein 1 (PD-1) inhibitor-based immunotherapy (pembrolizumab, nivolumab). Avelumab **is** approved for use in metastatic Merkel cell carcinoma in Australia

If chemotherapy is required. a regimen of a platinum compound plus etoposide is preferred.

Thus, in this comparison of drug availability for the treatment of non-melanoma skin cancer, two drugs approved in the USA – pembrolizumab and cemiplimab – are not yet approved for the respective indications in Australia.

Appendix A. Child-Pugh classification of hepatic impairment

Encephalopathy: None = 1 point, Grade 1 and 2 = 2 points, Grade 3 and 4 = 3 points

Ascites: None = 1 point, slight = 2 points, moderate = 3 points

Bilirubin: under 2 mg/ml = 1 point, 2 to 3 mg/ml = 2 points, over 3 mg/ml = 3 points

Albumin: greater than 3.5mg/ml = 1 point, 2.8 to 3.5mg/ml = 2 points, less than 2.8mg/ml = 3 points

Prothrombin Time* (sec prolonged): less than 4 sec = 1 point, 4 to 6 sec = 2 points, over 6 sec = 3 points

*Frequently INR will be used as a substitute for PT, with INR under 1.7 = 1 point, INR 1.7 to 2.2 = 2 points, INR above 2.2 = 3 points

The severity of cirrhosis:

Child-Pugh A: 5 to 6 points

Child-Pugh B: 7 to 9 points

Child-Pugh C: 10 to 15 points

Appendix B. **The grading of severity of adverse clinical and laboratory events**

From the U.S. DEPARTMENT OF HEALTH AND HUMAN SERVICES

Common Terminology Criteria for Adverse Events (CTCAE) Version 5.0 Published: November 27, 2017

This quick reference extensive document (155 pages) can be found at

https://ctep.cancer.gov/protocoldevelopment/electronic_applications/docs/CTCAE_v5_Quick_Reference_5x7.pdf

Appendix C. Definition of the cytokine response syndrome

From the USA National Cancer Institute:

A condition that may occur after treatment with some types of immunotherapy, such as monoclonal antibodies and CAR-T cells. Cytokine release syndrome is caused by a large, rapid release of cytokines into the blood from immune cells affected by the immunotherapy. Cytokines are immune substances that have many different actions in the body. Signs and symptoms of cytokine release syndrome include fever, nausea, headache, rash, rapid heartbeat, low blood pressure, and trouble breathing. Most patients have a mild reaction, but sometimes, the reaction may be severe or life threatening.

From Wikipedia (https://en.wikipedia.org/wiki/Cytokine_release_syndrome)

Cytokine release syndrome (CRS) is a form of systemic inflammatory response syndrome (SIRS) that can be triggered by a variety of factors such as infections and certain drugs. It refers to cytokine storm syndromes (CSS) and occurs when large numbers of white blood cells are activated and release inflammatory cytokines, which in turn activate yet more white blood cells. CRS is also an adverse effect of some monoclonal antibody medications, as well as adoptive T-cell therapies. When occurring as a result of a medication, it is also known as an infusion reaction.

The term cytokine storm is often used interchangeably with CRS but, despite the fact that they have similar clinical phenotype, their characteristics are different. When occurring as a result of a therapy, CRS symptoms may be delayed until days or weeks after treatment. Immediate-onset CRS is a cytokine storm, although severe cases of CRS have also been called cytokine storm

Symptoms include fever, fatigue, loss of appetite, muscle and joint pain, nausea, vomiting, diarrhea, rashes, fast breathing, rapid heartbeat, low blood pressure, seizures, headache, confusion, delirium, hallucinations, tremor, and loss of coordination.

Laboratory tests and clinical monitoring show low blood oxygen, widened pulse pressure, increased cardiac output (early), potentially diminished cardiac output (late), high levels of nitrogen compounds in the blood, elevated D-dimer, elevated transaminases, factor I deficiency and excessive bleeding, higher-than-normal level of bilirubin.

CRS occurs when large numbers of white blood cells, including B cells, T cells, natural killer cells, macrophages, dendritic cells, and monocytes are activated and release inflammatory cytokines, which activate more white blood cells in a positive feedback loop of pathogenic inflammation. Immune cells are activated by stressed or infected cells through receptor-ligand interactions.

This can occur when the immune system is fighting pathogens, as cytokines produced by immune cells recruit more effector immune cells such as T-cells and inflammatory monocytes (which differentiate into macrophages) to the site of inflammation or infection. In addition, pro-inflammatory cytokines binding their cognate receptor on immune cells results in activation and stimulation of further cytokine production. This process, when dysregulated, can be life-threatening due to systemic hyper-inflammation, hypotensive shock, and multi-organ failure.

Adoptive cell transfer of autologous T-cells modified with chimeric antigen receptors (CAR-T cell therapy) also causes CRS. Serum samples of patients with CAR-T associated CRS have elevated levels of IL-6, IFN-γ, IL-8 (CXCL8), IL-10, GM-CSF, MIP-1α/β, MCP-1 (CCL2), CXCL9, and CXCL10 (IP-10). The most predictive biomarkers 36h after CAR-T infusion of CRS are a fever ≥38.9 °C (102 °F) and elevated levels of MCP-1 in serum. Many of the cytokines elevated in CRS are not produced by CAR-T cells, but by myeloid cells that are pathogenically licensed through T-cell-mediated activating mechanisms. For example, in vitro co-culture experiments have demonstrated IL-6, MCP-1, and MIP-1 are not produced by CAR-T cells, but rather by inflammatory myeloid lineage cells. In vivo models have demonstrated NSG (NOD/SCID/γ-chain deficient mice) with defects of both lymphocyte and myeloid lineage compartments do not develop CRS after CAR-T cell infusion.

In addition to adoptive T-cell therapies, severe CRS or cytokine reactions can occur in a number of infectious and non-infectious diseases including graft-versus-host disease (GVHD), coronavirus disease 2019 (COVID-19), acute respiratory distress syndrome (ARDS), sepsis, Ebola, avian influenza, smallpox, and systemic inflammatory response syndrome (SIRS).

Although severe acute respiratory syndrome coronavirus 2 (SARS-CoV-2) is sufficiently cleared by the early acute phase anti-viral response in most individuals, some progress to a hyperinflammatory condition, often with life-threatening pulmonary involvement. This systemic hyperinflammation results in inflammatory lymphocytic and monocytic infiltration of the lung and the heart, causing ARDS and cardiac failure. Patients with fulminant COVID-19 and ARDS have classical serum biomarkers of CRS including elevated CRP, LDH, IL-6, and ferritin.

Hemophagocytic lymphohistiocytosis and Epstein-Barr virus-related hemophagocytic lymphohistiocytosis are caused by extreme elevations in cytokines and can be regarded as one form of severe cytokine release syndrome.

Medications

Cytokine reaction syndrome may also be induced by certain medications, such as the CD20 antibody rituximab and the CD19 CAR T cell tisagenlecleucel. The experimental drug TGN1412—also known as theralizumab—caused extremely serious symptoms when given to six participants in a Phase I trial. A controlled and limited CRS is triggered by active fever therapy with mixed bacterial vaccines (MBV) according to Coley; it is used for oncological and certain chronic diseases. CRS has also arisen with biotherapeutics intended to suppress or activate the immune system through receptors on white blood cells. Muromonab-CD3, an anti-CD3 monoclonal antibody intended to suppress the immune system to prevent rejection of organ transplants; alemtuzumab, which is anti-CD52 and used to treat blood cancers as well as multiple sclerosis and in organ transplants; and rituximab, which is anti-CD20 and used to treat blood cancers and auto-immune disorders, all cause CRS.

CRS needs to be distinguished from symptoms of the disease itself and, in the case of drugs, from other adverse effects—for example tumor lysis syndrome requires different interventions. As of 2015, differential diagnoses depended on the judgement of doctor as there were no objective tests.

CRS is a form of systemic inflammatory response syndrome and is an adverse effect of some drugs.

The Common Terminology Criteria for Adverse Events classifications for CRS as of version 4.03 issued in 2010 were:[5][20]

Grades	Toxicity
Grade 1	Mild reaction, infusion interruption not indicated; intervention not indicated
Grade 2	Therapy or infusion interruption indicated but responds promptly to symptomatic treatment (e.g., antihistamines, NSAIDS, narcotics, IV fluids); prophylactic medications indicated for <=24 hrs
Grade 3	Prolonged (e.g., not rapidly responsive to symptomatic medication or brief interruption of infusion); recurrence of symptoms following initial improvement; hospitalization indicated for clinical sequelae (e.g., renal

	impairment, pulmonary infiltrates)
Grade 4	Life-threatening consequences; pressor or ventilatory support indicated
Grade 5	Death

Appendix D. Cytokine storm

From Wikipedia (https://en.wikipedia.org/wiki/Cytokine_storm)

A cytokine storm, also called hypercytokinemia, is a physiological reaction in humans and other animals in which the innate immune system causes an uncontrolled and excessive release of pro-inflammatory signaling molecules called cytokines. Normally, cytokines are part of the body's immune response to infection, but their sudden release in large quantities can cause multisystem organ failure and death.

Cytokine storms can be caused by a number of infectious and non-infectious etiologies, especially viral respiratory infections such as H1N1 influenza, H5N1 influenza, SARS-CoV-1, and SARS-CoV-2, Influenza B, Parainfluenza virus, and Ebola. Other causative agents include the Epstein-Barr virus, cytomegalovirus, group A streptococcus, and non-infectious conditions such as graft-versus-host disease. The viruses can invade lung epithelial cells and alveolar macrophages to produce viral nucleic acid, which stimulates the infected cells to release cytokines and chemokines, activating macrophages, dendritic cells, and others.

Cytokine storm syndrome is a diverse set of conditions that can result in a cytokine storm. Cytokine storm syndromes include familial hemophagocytic lymphohistiocytosis, Epstein-Barr virus–associated hemophagocytic lymphohistiocytosis, systemic or non-systemic juvenile idiopathic arthritis–associated macrophage activation syndrome, NLRC4 macrophage activation syndrome, cytokine release syndrome and sepsis.

Cytokine storms versus cytokine release syndrome

The term "cytokine storm" is often loosely used interchangeably with cytokine release syndrome (CRS) but is more precisely a differentiable syndrome that may represent a severe episode of cytokine release syndrome or a component of another disease entity, such as macrophage activation syndrome. When occurring as a result of a therapy, CRS symptoms may be delayed until days or weeks after treatment. Immediate-onset (fulminant) CRS appears to be a cytokine storm.

Appendix E. Macrophage activation syndrome

From Wikipedia (https://en.wikipedia.org/wiki/Macrophage_activation_syndrome)

Macrophage activation syndrome is a severe, potentially life-threatening, complication of several chronic rheumatic diseases of childhood. It occurs most commonly with systemic-onset juvenile idiopathic arthritis (SoJIA). In addition, MAS has been described in association with systemic lupus erythematosus (SLE), Kawasaki disease, and adult-onset Still's disease. It is thought to be closely related and pathophysiologically very similar to reactive (secondary) hemophagocytic lymphohistiocytosis (HLH). The incidence of MAS is unknown as there is a wide spectrum of clinical manifestations, and episodes may remain unrecognized.

Signs and symptoms

The hallmark clinical and laboratory features include high fever, hepatosplenomegaly, lymphadenopathy, pancytopenia, liver dysfunction, disseminated intravascular coagulation, hypofibrinogenemia, hyperferritinemia, and hypertriglyceridemia. Despite marked systemic inflammation, the erythrocyte sedimentation rate (ESR) is paradoxically depressed, caused by low fibrinogen levels. The low ESR helps to distinguish the disorder from a flare of the underlying rheumatic disorder, in which case the ESR is usually elevated. A bone marrow biopsy or aspirate usually shows hemophagocytosis.

Cause

In many cases a trigger is identified, often a viral infection, or a medication. There is uncontrolled activation and proliferation of macrophages, and T lymphocytes, with a marked increase in circulating cytokines, such as IFN-gamma, and GM-CSF. The underlying causative event is unclear, and is the subject of ongoing research. In many cases of MAS, a decreased natural killer cell (NK-cell) function is found.

Diagnosis

A febrile patient with known or suspected sJia must be considered for macrophage activation if:

Ferritin >684 ng/ml

and any 2 of the following:

Hemoglobin <90g/L (in infants <4 weeks: <100g/L)

Platelets <100 x 109/L

Neutrophils <1.0 x 109/L

Fasting triglycerides ≥3.0 mmol/L (i.e., ≥ 265 mg/dl)

Fibrinogen ≤1.5 g/L[3]

In addition, other specific markers of macrophage activation (e.g. soluble CD163), and lymphocyte activation (e.g. soluble IL-2 receptor) can be helpful. NK cell function analysis may show depressed NK function, or, flow cytometry may show a depressed NK cell population.

Treatment

The best treatment for MAS has not been firmly established. Most commonly used treatments include high-dose glucocorticsteroids, and cyclosporine. In refractory cases treatment regimens are used similar to that in HLH.

Anakinra may also be effective.

Appendix F. Immune reconstitution inflammatory syndrome (IRIS)

From Wikipedia (https://en.wikipedia.org/wiki/Immune_reconstitution_inflammatory_syndrome)

Immune reconstitution inflammatory syndrome (IRIS) is a condition seen in some cases of AIDS or immunosuppression, in which the immune system begins to recover, but then responds to a previously acquired opportunistic infection with an overwhelming inflammatory response that paradoxically makes the symptoms of infection worse.

In HIV infection and immunosuppression

The suppression of CD4 T cells by HIV (or by immunosuppressive drugs) causes a decrease in the body's normal response to certain infections. Not only does this make it more difficult to fight the infection, it may mean that a level of infection that would normally produce symptoms is instead undetected (subclinical infection). If the CD4 count rapidly increases (due to effective treatment of HIV, or removal of other causes of immunosuppression), a sudden increase in the inflammatory response produces nonspecific symptoms such as fever, and in some cases a worsening of damage to the infected tissue.

There are two common IRIS scenarios. The first is the “unmasking” of an occult opportunistic infection. The second is the “paradoxical” symptomatic relapse of a prior infection despite microbiologic treatment success. Often in paradoxical IRIS, microbiologic cultures are sterile. In either scenario, there is hypothesized reconstitution of antigen-specific T cell-mediated immunity with activation of the immune system following HIV therapy against persisting antigen, whether present as intact organisms, dead organisms, or debris.

Though these symptoms can be dangerous, they also indicate that the body may now have a better chance to defeat the infection. The best treatment for this condition is unknown. In paradoxical IRIS reactions, the events will usually spontaneously get better with time without any additional therapy. In unmasking IRIS, the most common treatment is to administer antibiotic or antiviral drugs against the infectious organism. In some severe cases, anti-inflammatory medications, such as corticosteroids are needed to suppress inflammation until the infection has been eliminated.

Infections most commonly associated with IRIS include *Mycobacterium tuberculosis* and cryptococcal meningitis. Persons living with AIDS are more at risk for IRIS if they are starting HAART for the first time, or if they have recently been treated for an opportunistic infection (OI). It is generally advised that when patients have a low initial CD4 T cell count and opportunistic infection at the time of their HIV diagnosis, they receive treatment to control the opportunistic infections before

HAART is initiated approximately two weeks later. This is true for most OIs, except for OIs involving the central nervous system.

In cryptococcal meningitis

IRIS is particularly problematic in cryptococcal meningitis as IRIS is fairly common and can be fatal.

IRIS has been described in immunocompetent hosts who have meningitis caused by *Cryptococcus gattii* and *Cryptococcus neoformans var. grubii,* environmental fungi which often affect immunocompetent hosts. Several weeks or even months into appropriate treatment, there is a sudden onset deterioration with worsening meningitis symptoms and progression or development of new neurological symptoms.

Magnetic resonance imaging shows increase in the size of brain lesions, and CSF abnormalities (white cell count, protein, glucose) increase. CSF culture is typically sterile, and there is no increase in CSF cryptococcal antigen titer.

The increasing inflammation can cause brain injury or be fatal.

The general mechanism behind IRIS is increased inflammation as the recovering immune system recognizes the antigens of the fungus as immunosuppression is reversed. Cryptococcal IRIS has three phases:

- before HAART, with a paucity of cerebrospinal fluid (CSF) inflammation and defects in antigen clearance;
- during initial HAART immune recovery, with pro-inflammatory signaling by antigen-presenting cells without an effector response; and
- at IRIS, a cytokine storm with a predominant type-1 helper T cell interferon-gamma response.

Three clinical predictors of cryptococcal-related paradoxical IRIS risk include:

- lack of initial CSF pleocytosis (i.e. low CSF white blood cell count);
- elevated C-reactive protein;
- failure to sterilize the CSF before immune recovery.

IRIS may be the cause of paradoxically worse outcomes for cryptococcal meningitis in immunocompetent compared with immunocompromised hosts, in whom *Cryptococcus neoformans* is the usual pathogen. Treatment with systemic corticosteroids during IRIS may be beneficial in preventing death or progressive neurological deterioration. Corticosteroids given to persons with anti-fungal treatment failure / cryptococcal relapse (in whom CSF cultures are not sterile) can be a fatal iatrogenic error.

Glossary

Abbreviations used (other than those explained in Table1, Table 2 and in the FDA-derived text). This list includes abbreviations used in other books in the series Medicine 2020 and the series Modern Medicine 2021.

AC, adriamycin and cyclophosphamide (combination chemotherapy)

ACE, angiotensin-converting-enzyme

ADC, antibody-drug conjugate

ADCC, antibody-dependent cellular cytotoxicity

ADCC, antibody directed enzyme prodrug therapy

AGEP, acute generalized exanthematous pustulosis

AI, aromatase inhibitor

ALK, anaplastic lymphoma kinase

ALL, acute lymphoblastic leukemia

ALT, alanine aminotransferase

AML, acute myeloid leukemia

aPTT, activated partial thromboplastin time

ARR, administration-related reaction

AS, adverse reaction

AS, ankylosing spondylitis

ASCT, autologous stem cell transplant

AST, aspartate aminotransferase

ATA, anti-therapeutic antibody

ATM, ataxia telangiectasia mutated (gene)

AUC, Area Under the Concentration – time curve

AUC (0-inf): AUC curve to infinite time. As we cannot get the assays to go to infinity, we have to extrapolate to infinity. This can be calculated from the AUC(0-t) by the addition of a constant (Clast/λz), where Clast is the last observed quantifiable concentration and λz is the terminal phase rate constant.

BCG, Bacille Calmain-Guerin

BCR-ABL, breakpoint cluster region/Abelson

BCRP, breast cancer resistance protein

b DMARD, biologic disease-modifying anti-rheumatic drug

BRACA1, breast cancer susceptibility gene 1

BTK, Bruton's tyrosine kinase

CAT, cyclophosphamide, adriamycin and taxane (combination chemotherapy)

CDC, complement-dependent cytotoxicity

CDK, cyclin-dependent kinase

C-G, Cockoft-Gault (formula)

cHL, classical Hodgkin Lymphoma

CINV, chemotherapy-induced nausea and vomiting

CIS, carcinoma in situ

CLL, chronic lymphocytic leukemia

Clcr, creatinine clearance rate

CMF, cyclophosphamide, methotrexate, and fluorouracil (combination chemotherapy

CML, chronic myelogenous leukemia (also known as chronic myeloid leukemia)

CPS, combine positive score

CR, complete remission

CRC, colorectal carcinoma

CRS, cytokine release syndrome

CS, cytokine storm

csDMARD, synthetic disease-modifying anti-rheumatic drug

CSF1R, colony-stimulating factor receptor 1

CT, computed tomography

CTCAE, Common Terminology Criteria for Adverse Events

DCIS, ductal carcinoma in situ

DFS, disease-free survival

dMMR, deficient mismatch repair

DPP4, dipeptidyl peptidase-4

DRESS, drug reaction with eosinophilia and systemic symptoms. DRESS syndrome is classified as one form of severe cutaneous adverse reactions (SCARs). In addition to DRESS, SCARs includes four other drug-induced skin reactions, the Stevens–Johnson syndrome (SJS); Toxic epidermal necrolysis (TEN), Stevens–Johnson/toxic epidermal necrolysis overlap syndrome (SJS/TEN)

EBC, early breast cancer

ECG or EKG, electrocardiogram

EFS, event-free durvival

EGF, epidermal growth factor

EGFR, epidermal growth factor receptor

EN, erythema nodosum

ER, estrogen receptor

ET, endocrine therapy

ErbB, derived from erythroblastic leukemia viral oncogene

FBG, fasting blood glucose

FEC, fluorouracil, epirubicin and cyclophosphamide (combination chemotherapy)

FGF, fibroblast growth factor

FGFR, fibroblast growth factor receptor

FISH, fluorescence in situ hybridization

FKBP12/mTOR, FK Binding Protein-12/mammalian target of rapamycin

Flt3, fms like tyrosine kinase 3

FPG, fasting plams glucose

FSH, follicle-stimulating hormone

FU, fluouracil

gBRCAm, BRCA mutated

GD, gestational day

GI, gastro-intestinal

GIST, gastrointestinal stromal tumor

GFR, glomerular filtration rate

GMR, geometric mean ratio

HCC, hepatocellular carcinoma

HER, human epidermal receptor

HER2, human epidermal growth factor receptor 2

HNSCC, head and neck squamous carcinoma

HR, hormone receptor

HRR, homologous recombination repair

HSCT, hematopoietic stem cell transplant

JAK, Janus kinase

KLIFS-3, kinase-ligand interaction fingerprint and structure residue-3

IBC, inflammatory breast cancer

IC, immune cell

IFN, interferon

IL, interleukin

ILD, interstitial lung disease

ILN, interstitial lung disease

IRR, infusion-related reaction

ITP, idiopathic thrombocytopenic purpura

LCIS, lobular carcinoma in situ

LFT, lver function test

LH, luteinizing hormone

LLN, lower limit of normal

LVEF, left ventricular ejection fraction

Mab, monoclonal antibody

MATE, multi-antimicrobial extrusion protein

MBC, metastatic breast cancer

MCC, Merkel cell carcinoma

mCRPC, metastatic castrate resistant prostate cancer

MEK, mitogen-activated protein kinase

MRI, magnetic resonance imaging

MSI-H, microsatellite instability – high

MUGA, multigated acquisition

NCI-CTC, National Cancer Institute – Clinical Toxicity Criteria

Nib, small i**nhib**itory molecule

NMIBC, non-muscle invasive bladder cancer

NRH, nodular regenerative hyperplasia (of the liver)

NSCLC, non-small cell lung cancer

OS, overall survival

PARP, poly(ADP-ribose) polymerase

PDGF, platelet-derived growth factor

PDGFR, platelet-derived growth factor receptor

PFS, progression-free survival

Ph+, Philadelphia chromosome positive

PI3K, phosphatidylinositol 3-kinase

PI3KA, phosphatidylinositol-4,5-bisphosphate 3-kinase catalytic subunit alpha

PJIA, polyarticular juvenile idiopathic arthritis in patients aged 2 years or older

PJP, *Pneumocystis jiroveci* pneumonia

PK, pharmacokinetic analysis

PKA, protein kinase A

PMBCL, primary mediastinal B cell lymphoma

PNET, progressive neuroendocrine tumor (of the pancreasP

PR, progesterone receptor

pRb, retinoblastoma protein

PsA, psoriatic arthritis

PsO, plaque psoriasis

RA, rheumatoid arthritis

RAF, rapidly accelerated fibrosarcoma

RCC, renal cell carcinoma

RET, "rearranged during transfection”

ROCK, Rho-associated protein kinase

ROS, 'orphan' receptor tyrosine kinase

rb, retinoblastoma (gene or protein)

scFv, single-chain Fv fragment

SCARS, severe cutaneous adverse reactions

SCLC, small cell lung cancer

SERD, selective estrogen receptor degrader

SEGA, subependymal giant cell astrocytoma

SLAM, signalling lymphocytic activation molecule family (CD319)

SJS, Stevens–Johnson syndrome

SLL, small lymphocytic lymphoma

SYK, spleen tyrosine kinase

SWFI, sterile water for injection

TBC.tuberose sclerosid complex

TCH, docetaxel, carboplatin, and trastuzumab (combination chemotherapy)

TEN, toxic epidermal necrolysis

TNBC, triple negative breast cancer

TMB- high, tunor mutational burden - high

TNF, tumor necrosis factor

TRK, tropomyosin receptor kinase

ts DMARD, targeted synthetic disease-modifying anti-rheumatic drug

Tyk, tyrosine-protein kinase

UGT1A1, uridine diphosphate-glucuronosyl transferase 1A1

ULN, upper limit of normal

VEGF, vascular endothelial growth factor

VEGFR, vascular endothelial growth factor receptor

Made in the USA
Monee, IL
01 May 2026

49337677R00117